The New Public Health

The New Public Health

THE LIVERPOOL
EXPERIENCE

John Ashton and
Howard Seymour

OPEN UNIVERSITY PRESS
MILTON KEYNES · PHILADELPHIA

Open University Press
Celtic Court
22 Ballmoor
Buckingham MK18 1XW

and
1900 Frost Road, Suite 101
Bristol, PA19007, USA

First Published 1988. Reprinted 1990, 1991, 1992

British Library Cataloguing in Publication Data

Ashton, John, *1947-*
  The new public health.
  1. Public health
  I. Title II. Seymour, Howard
  614

  ISBN 0-335-15555-3
  ISBN 0-335-15550-2 Pbk

Library of Congress Cataloging-in-Publication Data

Ashton, John, 1947–
    New public health : the Liverpool experience / by John Ashton and
  Howard Seymour.
      p. cm.
    Bibliography: p.
    Includes index.
      1. Health promotion—England—Liverpool. 2. Public health—
  England—Liverpool. 3. Medical policy—England—Liverpool.
  I. Seymour, Howard. II. Title.
  RA488.L7A84 1988
  362.1′09427′53—dc19   88-15226 CIP
    ISBN 0-335-15555-3 ISBN 0-335-15550-2 (pbk.)

Typeset by Inforum Ltd, Portsmouth
Printed and bound in Great Britain by
Biddles Ltd, Guildford and King's Lynn

Contents

Preface

The world is a fast flowing river.

One of the most common parables told in relation to the New Public Health movement is that which equates health workers to life-savers standing beside a fast flowing river. Every so often a drowning person is swept alongside. The life-saver dives in to the rescue, retrieves the 'patient' and resuscitates them. Just as they have finished another casualty appears alongside. So busy and involved are the life-savers in all of this rescue work that they have no time to walk upstream and see why it is that so many people are falling in the river. What is necessary, it is argued, is to refocus upstream and what is needed generally among health workers is more 'upstream thinking'. Depending on your perspective you may be inclined to conclude that it is people themselves who are jumping in and that their sickness is their own fault, that they are being seduced or pushed into the river or that indeed all paths lead into the river, or that they are the victims of genuine accidents or acts of God.

Writing from Liverpool in 1988 it is clear that whatever your conclusions, whether as a member of the public or as a professional (not solely in the medical or social services), it is no longer enough to claim immunity from thought by virtue of being a life-saver, or in the case of members of the public, just trying to get on with daily life.

Fundamental changes are taking place both in the way we view ill-health and the way as individuals, families and governments we respond to it. In the United Kingdom ministerial reputations and careers are being made and lost out of the health-related issues of AIDS, drugs, heart disease and the environmental conditions of the inner cities. The once sacred National Health Service is under attack for failing to deliver the goods and the long assumed immunity to accountability of physicians is falling away week by week. In Liverpool, 26 per cent of adult men are unemployed and nationally the infant mortality rate has just risen for the first time in 16 years.

All of these facts are interconnected. A debate is underway for the hearts and minds of a generation. The outcome of that debate will have major consequences for the health of everybody, but especially for the socially disadvantaged. It is a debate which is not confined to the United Kingdom but is being enacted in one form or another throughout the world as part of a paradigm shift in the way in which we view health.

We hope that this book will contribute to the creative resolution of that debate. In many ways this is a parochial account, being based on work in one declining industrial region of Europe with a population of 2.5 million. On the other hand, the work which we have been involved with has brought us into direct contact with similar communities in many parts of the world and convinced us of the relevance of our experiences not only to the developed and post-developed, or fourth world, but also the third world.

This book is dedicated to Pam and Ellen and to our many friends around the world who will recognise mutual discussions, ideas and experiences in these pages.

John Ashton
Howard Seymour

1 Introduction: Medicine in Perspective

The Commonly Held View

Until quite recently it has been a commonly held view that all improvements in health are the results of scientific medicine. This view is based on people's own experience of the modern management of sickness by, in the most part, skilled and dedicated health workers and doctors who are able to draw on a wide and ever growing range of technical diagnostic procedures, potent medicines and sophisticated surgical interventions. The recent public memory until the advent of AIDS includes the apparent demise of epidemics of infectious disease, dramatic declines in maternal and infant mortality rates and the progressive increase in the proportion of the population living into old age. These trends coincided in Britain with the development of the National Health Service and, until recently, the availability to most people of good quality medical care when they needed it, at little or no immediate cost to themselves or their family. The assumption has tended to be that improvements in health were caused by the existence of a National Health Service.

This assumption has been reinforced by the advertising of pharmaceutical companies, by the popular image on television and in magazines and books of (male) doctors as romantic heroes, and by the very high level of faith which people have apparently had in their doctors. Clearly there have been advances in scientific medicine which have been of enormous benefit to millions of people, but has it really been the case that scientific medicine alone or even in the main part has been responsible for the dramatic improvements in mortality rates and life chances which have been evident in developed countries during the past 150 years? And what lesson does our understanding of how these improvements have been brought about hold for present-day efforts to improve health?

Limitations to the Commonly Held View

The majority of developed countries spend between 5 and 10 per cent of their gross national product on health services,*[1] most of this money being spent on hospital-based treatment for existing disease, the demand for which has no immediately apparent ceiling. At the time that the British National Health Service was established in 1948 there was a general belief that once the backlog of disease existing among the poor had been dealt with the costs of the service would reduce. This 'backlog' is now more accurately seen as an iceberg, or the outer layer of an onion. We have come to realize that the greater the material prosperity, the greater is the expectation of enjoying a good quality of health and the less our tolerance of anything which impedes it.

The National Health Service itself was largely based on a hospital network. Primary medical care from health centres was seen as being an important part of an integrated approach, but the financial situation in the late 1940s led to an early abandonment of the health centre programme. A health centre programme was for a time resurrected, but nevertheless only about one-quarter of general practitioners currently work from such a centre and the continuing priority accorded to hospital medicine is manifested by the relative shift of resources away from preventive medicine and primary care into the hospital sector during the past 40 years. Between 1950 and 1981 the proportion of expenditure allocated to hospital services increased from 55 to 62 per cent, while that on General Practice declined from 10 to 6.5 per cent, and that on Health Authority Community Services from 8 to 6.5 per cent. There have been recent attempts to redress the balance, particularly in relation to such policies as that of closing long-stay institutions for the mentally ill and handicapped and resettling residents in small community units, but at a time of a restricted overall budget and the growing demands of an ageing population the inherent inertia which militates against moving budgets between programme areas is reinforced.

It has become clear to governments of all political persuasions in many countries that the demand for treatment services is limitless and cost-containment is now a priority in systems based on private health care linked to insurance as well as state-funded national health services. In the ensuing reappraisal, the cost-effectiveness of prevention compared with cure has become ever more emphasized, and it has been forcefully argued that too much emphasis is being placed on medical treatment and attempts at cure and insufficient on prevention (Fig. 1.1). Such sentiments have led to attempts to define the scope for prevention and to achieve a shift in emphasis away from treatment.[2,3]

The McKeown Hypothesis

One of the most influential voices in this debate has been that of Thomas McKeown, former Professor of Social Medicine at Birmingham. McKeown

---

* Superscript numerals refer to numbered references at the end of each chapter.

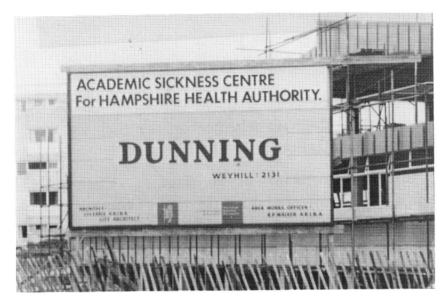

Fig. 1.1.   Health service or sickness service?

produced a synthesis of ideas for a new public health, based on an historical analysis of the reasons for the growth of the population in England and Wales and reflecting ideas from such as Sigerist, Ryle and Morris.[4–8]

The population of England and Wales in 1086 was of the order of 1.25 million, as estimated from the *Domesday Book*.[9] For the next 600 years there was a slow overall growth, interrupted by dramatic declines as a consequence of the plague (Black Death), which may have reduced the population by anything up to one-half in 1348–9.[10] By 1695 the population stood at about 5.5 million.

Accurate figures are available from the decennial census that has been conducted since 1801 when the population was nearly 9 million (Fig. 1.2). The population doubled in the first half of the nineteenth cenury and nearly doubled again in the second half. Since 1901 the increase has slowed and has now stopped, the most recent period having been marked by dramatic reductions in the overall size of birth cohorts of between 25 and 30 per cent, deferment of the birth of first children and a marked trend towards one- or two-child families.

The possible explanations for a change in population size include a positive balance of immigration, an increase in the birth rate or a decline in the death rate. Migration does not appear to have been an important factor and it is unlikely that the population increase before the middle of the nineteenth century was caused by an increasing birth rate. This was already high and had, in fact, begun to decline in the latter part of the century. McKeown has argued that the dramatic increase in population is to be accounted for by a

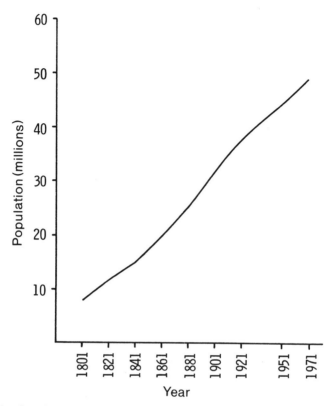

Fig. 1.2. Population of England and Wales at the time of the decennial censuses, 1801–1971.

reduction in death rates, especially in childhood (Fig. 1.3).

As a consequence the expectation of life at birth has increased considerably, and in the technologically advanced countries more than 95 per cent of the population survives to adult life. There has been a much smaller increase in life expectation at older ages. The overall effect of reduced birth rates and greater survival has been a major change in population structure, such that 4 per cent of the population was of retirement age in 1900, 16 per cent today and a projected 20 per cent plus by the year 2000 (males aged 65 and females aged 60). Likewise, we are about to witness a large increase in the very old (over 75) from 6 per cent in 1981 to 7 per cent by the year 2000; the over-75s currently consume many times more medical and social services than the under-75s.

During most of the existence of the human race it is probable that a large proportion of all children died or were killed in the first few years of life. However, the decline in death rates which began in the eighteenth century has continued until the present time, and in a careful analysis of the causes of death

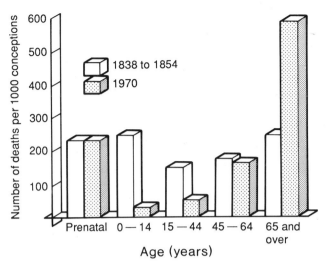

Fig. 1.3. Death rates per 1000 conceptions at various ages in England and Wales (after McKeown, 1976).

McKeown has concluded that the high death rates of the past were to a large extent attributable to a combination of infectious diseases with nutritional and other environmental factors. McKeown has estimated that between 80 and 90 per cent of the total reduction in the death rate from the beginning of the eighteenth century to the present day has been caused by a reduction in those deaths caused by infection. The most important of these have been tuberculosis, chest infections and the water- and food-borne diarrhoeal diseases which between them accounted for about half of the total reduction in deaths over this period.

McKeown considers that the predominance of infectious diseases probably dates from the first agricultural revolution when people first began to congregate in populations of considerable size. This was initially accompanied by a reduced mortality rate, occasioned by increased food production and increased numbers to the point at which starvation and malnutrition produced populations which were at risk for epidemics, especially air-borne ones. Increases in nutritional status then became necessary for substantial and prolonged falls in mortality and this occurred in the eighteenth and nineteenth centuries. From the second half of the nineteenth century, these trends were supported by a reduction in the exposure to infections as a result of their reduced prevalance and improved hygiene, i.e. higher food, water and housing standards.

The Contribution of Immunization and Therapy

McKeown's analysis is striking for its conclusion that with the exception of vaccination against smallpox, which was associated with less than 2 per cent of the decline in the death rate from 1848 to 1871, it is unlikely that immunization or therapy had a significant effect on mortality from infectious diseases before the twentieth century. In particular, most of the reduction in mortality from tuberculosis, bronchitis, pneumonia and influenza, whooping cough and food- and water-borne diseases had already occurred before effective immunization or treatment was available. Between 1900 and 1935 some specific measures contributed to reductions in death rates from infection. These included antitoxin in diphtheria, surgery in appendicitis, peritonitis, ear infections, salvarsan in syphilis, intravenous therapy in diarrhoeal disease, passive immunization against tetanus and improved obstetric care. However, the total contribution of medical and surgical interventions to reductions of mortality has been small compared with the impact of environmental 'public health', political, economic and social measures.

The Changing Importance of Non-infectious Diseases

Before the twentieth century infanticide and starvation were among the more common non-infectious hazards to life which have since almost disappeared in England and Wales. The largest fall in mortality between 1901 and 1971 was accounted for by conditions related to premature and immature birth and other diseases of infancy. Contributing factors have included better maternal nutrition, thereby reducing the incidence of premature birth, and better birth control and legal abortion resulting, initially, in a more planned spacing of children, with the benefit to mothers that they were able to recover from one pregnancy before falling pregnant again and to infants through extending the period of breast feeding and thereby increasing resistance to infectious disease. These effects have led to reductions in both maternal and child mortality rates. More recently there have been dramatic changes in family size associated with the changing expectations of women and of society generally. Improved obstetric care and management of the premature infant are comparatively recent additions which have helped to consolidate historically very low mortality rates.

McKeown[4] concluded from his analysis that:

> in order of importance the major contributions to improvements in health in England and Wales were from limitation of family size (a behavioural change), increase in food supplies and a healthier physical environment (environmental influences) and specific preventive and therapeutic measures.

It is clear from McKeown's work that in the past the impact of medicine has been more on disability than on death, and that: 'past improvement has been due mainly to modification of behaviour and changes in the environment and it is to these same influences that we must look for further advance'. The rational approach would appear to be to tackle those behavioural and environmental factors and their determinants which affect health in the twentieth century with the same vigour and determination that was applied to their predecessors in the nineteenth century. While not minimizing the value of clinical medicine, especially in reducing the consequences of those diseases which cannot be prevented, it is important to realize that medical care is but one factor in determining the health of a population.

Defining the Problem

In 1986 the infant mortality rate for England and Wales was 9.6 per 1000.[11] This compares with infant mortality rates of the last century which were commonly in excess of 100 per 1000. As recently as 1970, the rate within the Mersey Region, based on Liverpool, was 21 per 1000. Of great worry is the fact that the 1986 rate has increased for the first time in 16 years, presumably indirectly reflecting the deteriorating economic and social conditions of those living in poverty in Britain in the 1980s.

The expectation of life for males surviving to their first birthday in England and Wales is now 71 years and for females is 77 years. In developed countries it is now commonly considered abnormal for people to die before they reach old age.

A great deal still needs to be done in ensuring that the conditions of pregnancy and early life are optimal for the production of healthy, surviving infants and, in particular, in removing quite gross continuing geographical and social class inequalities. From a national point of view, England and Wales, for example, still have some way to go to be on a par with a number of other European countries (Table 1.1). A large part of the remaining infant deaths are accounted for by congenital disorders in the first weeks of life for which there are no immediate prospects of prevention. At the moment, all that we can offer is that for some of these conditions, notably Downs Syndrome and spina bifida together with some of the rare inherited disorders of biochemistry, it is possible to screen women during pregnancy and to offer an abortion to

Table 1.1   Infant mortality rate per 1000 live- and still-births in Europe

Country	1960	1978	% change 1960–78
Sweden	16.6	7.8	−53
Switzerland	21.1	8.6	−59
Denmark	21.5	8.6	−59
England and Wales	21.8	13.1	−40
France	27.4	10.6	−61
Belgium	31.2	13.9	−55
Luxembourg	31.5	8.1	−74

those found to be affected – where this is ethically acceptable to those women involved. Nevertheless, the systematic application of our current knowledge of human genetics through genetic counselling and screening should be a priority and investment in genetic research is likely to reap benefits during the next two or three decades.

Years of Lost Life

The declining usefulness of death rates for making assessments of a community's health has led to a search for other indicators. One such indicator is that of years of life lost before an assumed hypothetical natural life-span has been run. Such an approach serves to highlight the importance of causes of death in early life as each death carries with it a commensurately greater number of lost years. In particular, it stresses the importance of genetic causes, accidents and the smoking-related diseases of the heart and lungs. As indicators of death have declined in importance so have indicators of the quality of life been sought. Attention has increasingly been focussed on measures of physical, emotional and social ill-health to define need and assist in the evaluation of health and social policies and services. There have been many attempts to define 'health' in useful ways including the World Health Organization (WHO) definition of 'A complete state of physical, mental and social well-being and not merely the absence of disease.'[12] Although this definition has been criticized as being an impossible goal which cannot be translated into operational terms, some ultimate vision is probably necessary.

More recently, the World Health Organization has identified a more tangible definition in keeping with the WHO *Global Strategy of Health For All by the Year 2000* (HFA 2000).[3] The goal of HFA 2000 is that:

> the main social target of governments and WHO in the coming decades should be the attainment by all citizens of the world by the year 2000 of a level of health that will permit them to lead a socially and economically productive life.

Clearly such an approach recognizes and accepts both that healthy minds and healthy bodies go together and that health is a social rather than a narrowly biological or medical concept. It also recognizes the importance of useful and satisfying work in the well-being of individuals and of their communities. Some aspects of this perspective are touched on in the suggestion that health should be viewed as the 'foundation of achievement'.[14]

The Determinants of Health

Medical care, whether organized and professional or derived from family and friends as self-care, can only underpin the health of communities when prevention fails and as the means of support as biological systems run down in old age. Genetic endowment, environmental, nutritional, occupational and life-style factors must all be considered in any comprehensive approach to health.

GENETIC ENDOWMENT

The fundamental starting point for a consideration of the health of a population is the genetic endowment of its members. Genetic disorders are rarely susceptible to cure and often the best that can be offered is genetic counselling once a woman has given birth to an affected child. In relative terms, genetic abnormality is now responsible for a very sizeable proportion of the residual mortality and morbidity of newborn babies as other causes such as infection and malnutrition have been removed. Although the genetic factors which determine our biological potential at birth are much better understood than even 20 years ago, this area of knowledge remains one of the great frontiers for research which have major implications for preventive medicine.

In the meantime, of the 30,000 births annually in the Mersey Health Region 300 children are born suffering from major abnormalities which could have been detected during pregnancy and their mothers offered selective abortion. These include cases of Downs Syndrome, spina bifida and anencephaly, and a number of rarer chromosome disorders.

ENVIRONMENTAL FACTORS

Traditional environmental considerations concerning air, water, food, hygiene and shelter remain of major concern particularly in the context of a declining economy, and to these traditional considerations have been added new ones as a result of changing knowledge, expectations and technologies. Aesthetic, psychological and social considerations are now essential parts of any approach to the establishment of new standards rather than solely a consideration of the protection of physical health. There is a growing awareness of the ecological dimension and recognition of the indivisibility of life-style and habitat in relation to health.

NUTRITIONAL FACTORS

Historically the problem of nutrition was one of periodic inadequacy of food supplies. For many people on the margins of poverty such considerations remain real enough today. The new poor are the unemployed, especially those from ethnic minorities, single-parent families, the chronic sick and many pensioners. In addition, as described in the recent report by the National

Advisory Committee on Nutrition Education (NACNE), the nation's diet has in some ways changed for the worse since the war as a consequence of economic, technological and social developments.[18]

OCCUPATIONAL HEALTH

Occupational health in many countries continues to be a neglected area. New initiatives and a systematic approach are indicated. The counterpart of occupational health today is a concern for the health of the army of unemployed who constitute a major group at risk for a variety of health problems.

LIFE-STYLE

Life-style as a determinant of health is currently attracting a great deal of attention because, increasingly, it is unhealthy behaviours established as habits and sustained over long periods which can be pin-pointed as major avoidable health risks.

Medical Care – Formal and Informal

There is a growing recognition of the importance of good-quality, team-based primary medical care as the basis of a comprehensive system of medical care which also concerns itself with prevention. It has now become apparent that we have neglected the importance of self-care as an essential part of the medical care system. The medicalization of large areas of life has tended to undermine the role of individuals and social groups as partners in the process of maintaining and improving the health of the community. The women's movement has been instrumental in reviving an interest in self-care and self-help. The danger is that it can be seen as a cheap substitute to professionally provided care, rather than being a socially creative addition to it and part of the process of achieving a real participation in health.

In recent years it has become clear, particularly through the publication of the Black Report on inequalities in health in England and Wales, that all six of these determinants of health are strongly linked to social class, sex, race and geography within the United Kingdom.[19]

Inequalities in Health

Even when medical care seems to be relevant and of value it has become clear from the British experience that organized health services may not be responsive to needs in the way which one might have wished. There is now considerable evidence of what has been called an 'inverse care law', namely that those most in need of services are those least likely to receive them and vice versa.[15,16] Further, there is a well-recognized tendency throughout the world for the best qualified professional workers to themselves work among the middle classes rather than those most in need.

The Black Report documented the inequalities that exist in the mortality experience of men and women between the different social classes in different parts of the country and between different racial groups. This report has become a model for similar analyses in many other countries, both at a national and local level.[19]

The working party which produced the Black Report under the chairmanship of Sir Douglas Black, President of the Royal College of Physicians of England, had as their terms of reference 'to review information about differences in health status between the social classes, to consider possible causes and to suggest further research'. The working group faced a formidable task in bringing together large amounts of data from widely disparate sources and they sought information from other countries to the extent that it was available. A great deal of the information that they would have liked to have had just did not exist and it was not feasible for them to carry out special studies in the time available to them. Their task was not made any easier by the lack of commitment to the working group following the change of National Government in 1979; and when the report was published in the summer of 1980 the handling of it by the government was highly atypical for government publications. In fact, the report which appeared was a poor, photocopied draft of which only 200 copies were initially produced and distributed through an obscure Department of Health address rather than through the government stationery office as is customary. It was later held by critics that the government's handling of the report, which included a release date during Bank Holiday week, was intended to minimize the publicity which the report would receive. In the brief and curt introduction the Secretary of State for Health effectively rejected the report as unrealistic.

The Black Report

Far from disappearing in a sea of disinterest the Black Report continues to produce a wide-ranging debate on the causes of inequalities in health. There is little doubt that the report itself has achieved the status of a major reference document in the genre of Chadwick's report of the Committee of Inquiry into the Sanitary Conditions of the Labouring Population, which was published in 1842 and provided a good deal of background for the first Public Health Act of 1848.[20]

The Black Report, like Chadwick's, has brought together in one place information which cannot be politically ignored indefinitely. It shows clearly that major differences exist in the environmental factors which impinge on health, in the personal risk factors relating to life-style and in access to and use of preventive and treatment services. Above all, the report singles out the concentration of severe inequalities in 10 of the 200 British Health Districts.

SEX AND SOCIAL CLASS

Using the conventional Registrar General's classification of occupation as a proxy for social class, men of all social classes were found to have higher mortality rates than women of the same class, and there was a marked social class gradient in mortality rates for both men and women, with skilled and unskilled workers having higher rates than professionals.

GEOGRAPHY

Again using mortality as an indicator of ill-health, the healthiest part of Britain was confirmed to be the southern belt below the line drawn from the Wash to the Bristol Channel. The standardized mortality ratios, corrected for age and social class differences, reveal a range of 90 in the South-East to 113 in the North (England and Wales = 100; the North-East = 105). This is a variation of 26 per cent between highest and lowest.

ETHNIC ORIGIN

Statistics of mortality rates by country of birth and occupational class reveal a more complicated picture with low rates for manual skilled and unskilled immigrants but higher rates in the professions. The reasons for this are unclear.

The 'Black Working Party' found that manual workers were at a notable disadvantage in several respects, including:

1. The proportion giving birth to low birth weight infants.
2. Still-birth rates and death rates in the first year of life.
3. Greatly increased risk of accidental death in childhood and adult life.
4. Death from a wide variety of causes including cancers, heart and respiratory diseases.
5. Longstanding illness and restricted activity rates caused by disability.

One of the most disturbing findings was that disparities between the social classes have been increasing over the past 30 years.

When it comes to the availability and use of health services it seems that:

1. Children of professional parents make relatively greater use of general practitioner services than do children of manual workers.
2. Working-class women are much more likely than their professional sisters to book late for antenatal care and to make less use for themselves and their children of a range of preventive health services including dentistry, immunization and screening for cancer of the cervix.
3. Working-class pensioners are less likely to have their needs for chiropody

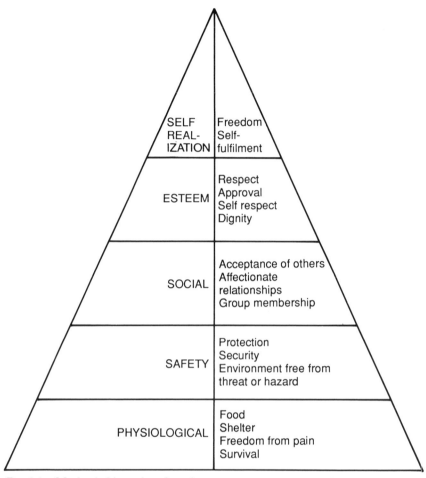

Fig. 1.4.   Maslow's hierarchy of needs.

met (and, presumably, of other similar services). With respect to personal risk factors, working-class men and women tend to smoke more, exercise less and to eat the types of food which now seem to be incriminated in diseases of the heart, blood vessels and bowel. Sir Douglas Black's group concluded that the most powerful explanation of the social class difference which they found was that which related them to material deprivation and poverty. Such a view is in keeping with common sense and accords with Maslow's hierarchy of needs which begin with the physical necessities of life (Fig. 1.4). Survival itself is necessary before people can hope to begin to realize their full potential, both psychological and social as well as physical.[21]

The need to take a holistic integrated view of health becomes clear.

References

1. Maxwell, R. (1974). *Health Care – The Growing Dilemma*. McKinsey and Co., New York.
2. HMSO (1979). *Prevention and Health: Everybody's Business*. HMSO, London.
3. HMSO (1977). *First Report from the Expenditure Committee. Preventive Medicine*. HMSO, London.
4. McKeown, T. (1976). *The role of Medicine – Dream, Mirage or Nemesis*. Nuffield Provincial Hospitals Trust, London.
5. Sigerist, H. (1941). *Medicine and Human Welfare*. Oxford University Press, Oxford.
6. Ryle, J.A. (1948). *Changing Disciplines*. Oxford University Press, Oxford.
7. Morris, J.N. (1975). *Uses of Epidemiology*. Churchill Livingstone, Edinburgh.
8. Morris, J.N. (1980). Are health services important to the peoples health? *British Medical Journal* **280**: 167–8.
9. Cartwright, F.F. (1977). *A Social History of Medicine*. Longmans, London.
10. Waters, W.E. (1977). Matters of Life and Death. Inaugural Lecture, University of Southampton, Southampton.
11. Office of Populations Censuses and Surveys (1986). *1986 Vital Statistics*. OPCS, London.
12. World Health Organization (1946). *Constitution*. WHO, Geneva.
13. World Health Organization (1981). *Global Strategy for Health For All by the Year 2000*. WHO, Geneva.
14. Seedhouse, D. (1986). *Health – The Foundations of Achievement*. John Wiley, New York.
15. Townsend, P. (1974). Inequality and the Health Service. *Lancet* **i**, 1179–90.
16. Tudor Hart, J. (1971). The Inverse Care Law. *Lancet* **i**, 405–12.
17. Chambers, R. (1983). *Rural Development: Putting the Last First*. Longmans, London.
18. NACNE (1983). *Proposals for Nutritional Guidelines for Health Education in Britain*. Health Education Council, London.
19. Townsend, P. and Davidson, N. (1982). *Inequalities in health – The Black Report*. Penguin, Harmondsworth.
20. Chadwick, E. (1842). *The Sanitary Condition of the Labouring Population of Great Britain*. Republished (1965, ed. M.W. Flinn) by Edinburgh University Press, Edinburgh.
21. Maslow, A.H. (1968). *Towards A Psychology of Being*. Van Nostrand Reinhold, New York.

2 The Setting for a New Public Health

In Europe and North America three distinct phases of activity in relation to public health can be identified in the last 150 years.[1] The first phase began in the industrialized cities of Northern Europe in response to the appalling toll of death and disease among the working classes living in abject poverty. The displacement of large numbers of people from the land by their landlords in order to take advantage of the agricultural revolution had combined with the attraction of the growing cities as the result of the industrial revolution to produce a massive change in population patterns and in the physical environments in which people lived.[2-6] The predominantly rural ecology of human habitation was ruptured and replaced by one in which a seething mass of humanity was living in squalor.

In Liverpool, which was the first city to appoint a medical officer of health, Dr Duncan, the population of what had been little more than a fishing village in 1650 reached 60,000 by 1770, and 120,000 by 1820; this rate of growth was sustained for another 100 years so that the population peaked at about 900,000 in the 1930s (Fig. 2.1 and 2.2). Duncan, who was working as a general practitioner in the central area of Liverpool in the 1830s, became so concerned at the housing conditions of his parents that he carried out a survey. He discovered that one-third of the population was living in the cellars of back-to-back houses with earth floors, no ventilation or sanitation and as many as 16 people to a room. It was not surprising, he maintained, that 'the fevers were rampant', that the epidemics of crowd diseases such as tuberculosis, pneumonia, whooping cough, measles and smallpox flourished under such conditions. Nor was it surprising that cholera which is normally water-borne should assume the contagious characteristics of these diseases under such conditions (Fig. 2.3 and 2.4).[4,7] The response to this situation was the gradual development of a public health movement based on the activities of medical officers of health, sanitary inspectors and their staff, supported by legislation such as the local Liverpool Sanitary Act of 1846 and the National Public Health Acts of 1848 and 1875 in England.[7]

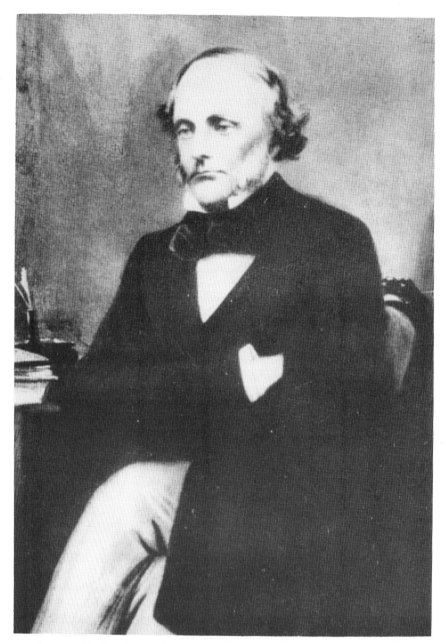

Fig. 2.1.   Dr William Henry Duncan, first Medical Officer of Health.

The focus of this movement was improvements in housing and sanitation standards and the provision of bacteriologically safe water and food. A specific example of the kind of measures taken was the establishment of the first public

Population
(thousands)

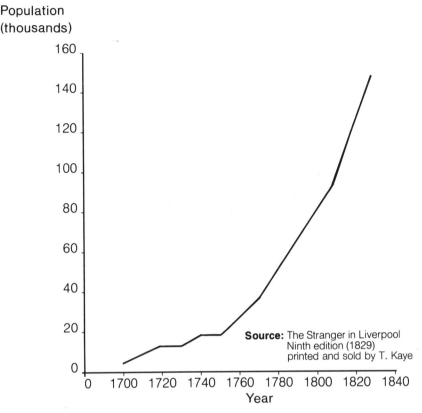

Fig. 2.2.   The growth of population in Liverpool, 1700–1829.

wash-house in the world which was opened in Liverpool in 1842 (Fig. 2.5).

The Public Health Movement with its emphasis on environmental change lasted until the 1870s and was in time eclipsed by a more individualistic approach ushered in by the development of the germ theory of disease and the possibilities offered by immunization and vaccination. As the most pressing environmental problems were brought under control, action to improve the health of the population moved on first to personal preventive medical services, such as immunization and family planning, and later to a range of other initiatives including the development of community and school nursing and school health services, again pioneered in Liverpool perhaps more from necessity than from inspiration. The introduction of school meals came as part of a package of measures to try and do something about the poor conditions of working-class recruits to the army, during the Boer War at the turn of the century.[8,9] That it was possible to contemplate school-based measures at all was a result of the extension of education following the 1870 Education Act. The second phase also marked the increasing involvement of the State in

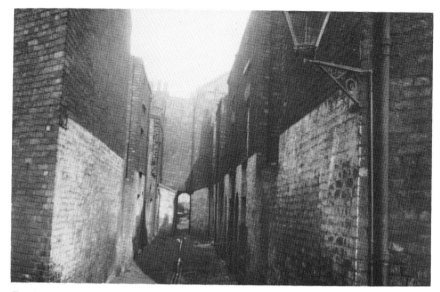

Fig. 2.3.   Typical back-to-back housing in Liverpool dating from the early nineteenth century.

medical and social welfare through the provision of hospital and clinic services.[10]

The second phase was in its turn superseded by the therapeutic era, dating from the 1930s, with the advent of insulin and the sulphonamide group of drugs. Until that time there was little of proven efficacy in the therapeutic arsenal.[2] The beginning of this era coincided with the apparent demise of infectious diseases on the the one hand and the development of ideas about the welfare state in many developed countries on the other. Historically, it marked a weakening of departments of public health and a shift of power and resources to hospital-based services and particularly those based in teaching hospitals.

Despite the outstanding work of many public health practitioners, in this process the imperative of population coverage which underpins public health rather than concern for individuals who are able to pay for a service has not always been to the fore as evidenced by the continuing and widening inequalities in health.[11-13] This may have something to do with the relative nature of infectious and non-infectious disease and their impact on governing élites – in order to protect themselves from infectious disease it is necessary for the middle-classes to ensure that the whole population is protected, whereas this may not be the case with non-infectious diseases.

It seems probable that when the Victorian cholera epidemics affected the middle-class areas of the great cities, the argument against paying for public health out of the rates was quickly lost.[14] Similarly, the contemporary problems of drug abuse and AIDS which are no respecters of social class have produced dramatic and costly government responses in many countries.

By the early 1970s the therapeutic era was increasingly being challenged.

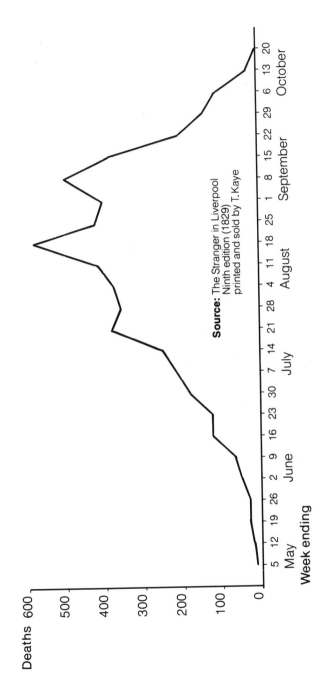

Source: The Stranger in Liverpool
Ninth edition (1829)
printed and sold by T.Kaye

Deaths 600 500 400 300 200 100 0

5 12 19 26 2 9 16 23 30 7 14 21 28 4 11 18 25 1 8 15 22 29 6 13 20

May June July August September October

Week ending

Fig. 2.4. Weekly deaths from cholera in Liverpool in 1829.

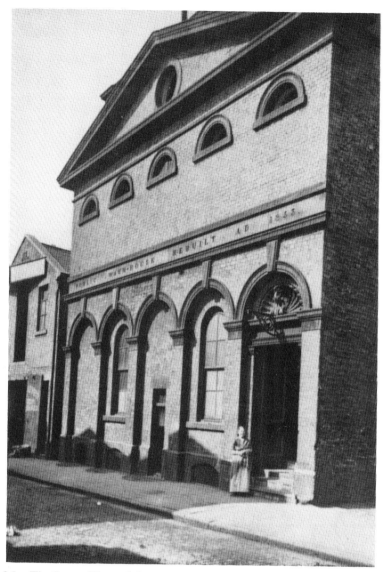

Fig. 2.5.　The first public wash-house in the world opened in Upper Frederick Street, Liverpool in 1842.

Most countries were experiencing a crisis in health care costs irrespective of their structure of health services; the escalation in costs being in part consequent on technological innovation in treatment methods and an apparently limitless demand for medical care, coupled with the dramatic demographic changes which were taking place with very rapid growth of the elderly population. McKeown's analysis, together with root and branch critiques of medical practice, such as that of Ivan Illich, lent support to the growing interest in a reappraisal of priorities.[2,15]

Illich had argued in effect that far from being part of the solution the activities of the medical profession were part of the problem; i.e. in its way of functioning, modern medicine had not only taken away from people the control over their own bodies and health but was actually responsible for a great deal of iatrogenic disease. Such a view was reinforced by the growth of feminist ideas, experiments with alternative life-styles and the treatments and attempts to reclaim health as a legitimate area for lay- and self-help.[16–18]

In 1974, the then Canadian Minister of Health, Marc Lalonde, published a government report entitled *A New Perspective on the Health of Canadians*. This report, which was a community diagnosis for Canada, focussed attention on the fact that a great deal of premature death and disability in Canada was preventable.[19] In effect it set an agenda for a new era of preventive medicine in Canada; it is arguable that it signalled the turning point in efforts to rediscover public health in developed countries and that it ushered in a new, fourth phase of public health.

What is emerging as the New Public Health is an approach which brings together environmental change and personal preventive measures with appropriate therapeutic interventions, especially for the elderly and disabled. However, the New Public Health goes beyond an understanding of human biology and recognizes the importance of those social aspects of health problems which are caused by life-styles. In this way it seeks to avoid the trap of blaming the victim. Many contemporary health problems are therefore seen as being social rather than solely individual problems; underlying them are concrete issues of local and national public policy, and what are needed to address these problems are 'Healthy Public Policies' – policies in many fields which support the promotion of health.[20–23] In the New Public Health the environment is social and psychological as well as physical.

Since 1974, many countries have published similar prevention-orientated documents and there has been an explosion of interest in preventive medicine and health promotion.[24,25] In this growing movement an important lead has been provided by the work of the World Health Organization.

Health For All by the Year 2000

The increasing momentum and desire for a new public health movement to tackle the health problems of the twenty-first century found its expression in the World Health Organization's *Global Strategy of Health For All by the Year 2000 (HFA 2000)*, which was accepted as WHO policy in 1981 by the thirty-fourth World Health Assembly. According to this strategy the task is to ensure that by the year 2000:

all people in all countries should have at least such a level of health that they are capable of working productively and of participating actively in the social life of the community in which they live.

The development of primary health care is seen as being central to the attainment of the goal of HFA 2000 and it is recognized that the strategy depends on the development of real community participation and collaboration between different sectors and agencies (intersectoral collaboration).[27]

In their strategy document, WHO identifies three main objectives for health for all in addition to these overriding principles:

- Promotion of life-styles conducive to health.
- Prevention of preventable conditions.
- Rehabilitation and health services.

These objectives have been further clarified in ways which make it possible for health goals to be set. Within Europe, the World Health Organization Regional Office has developed its own strategy for health for all which has been endorsed by all 33 member states.[28]

THE PROMOTION OF LIFE-STYLES CONDUCIVE TO HEALTH

1. The development of individual awareness of health risks and the changes in behaviour needed to improve health. This must be developed early in life.
2. Intersectoral approaches through both government and the wider institutions of the community are needed to improve social and economic conditions which influence choice of life-style. These conditions include job opportunities, working and living conditions and social networks.
3. Health risks which are to some extent self-imposed, such as alcohol and other drug dependencies, smoking, unbalanced nutrition, sexually transmitted diseases, unintended pregnancies and other disruptive elements of life-style can be reduced by information and education. However, they need to be supported by healthy public policies which help 'to make the Healthy Choices the Easy Choices'; this may involve legislative and regulatory controls.

PREVENTION OF PREVENTABLE CONDITIONS

1. Mothers and children are identified as a priority group. Priority services should include adequate primary care, including perinatal, maternal, infant and child care, and genetic counselling with facilities for family planning and abortion when needed. Emphasis should be put on comprehensive early detection of defects and risk factors.
2. To reduce the incidence of the remaining communicable diseases all

children should be covered by appropriate immunization programmes by 1990.
3. More strenuous efforts are needed to reduce accidents and their consequences. These include innovative approaches to public health education, road design and construction and traffic regulation, safety at work, in the home and during recreation and the design of vehicles and consumer goods.
4. Education to discourage obesity and encourage balanced nutrition and breast-feeding and food safety regulations.
5. The provision of safe water and sanitation.

REHABILITATION AND HEALTH SERVICES

1. All people should have access to community-based primary health care which gives priority to preventive medicine and health promotion and supports self-help and self-care with greater attention being given to the humanization of health services.
2. Special services for underserved and high-risk groups such as the elderly, mentally ill, mentally handicapped and disabled.
3. There should be earlier diagnosis and intervention to prevent the establishment of chronic and degenerative disease.
4. There should be improvements in the quality and cost-effectiveness of services as well as in the equity of provision.

The key elements of this strategy are that it is aimed at the elimination of inequalities in health and that it is based on a broad, public health concept of primary care.

It is the underlying intention of the 'Health For All Strategy' that each country and region within countries should develop its own health for all strategy. This has begun to happen to some extent in Europe and, importantly, the member states have agreed a set of 38 targets with appropriate indicators as steps on the path to health for all (Table 2.1).[29]

The European programme is intended to achieve a shift away from a narrow medical view through an expansion in five areas.

1. Self-care.
2. Integration of medical care with other related activities such as education, recreation, environmental improvements and social welfare (so-called intersectoral action).
3. Integrating the promotion of good health with preventive medicine, treatment and rehabilitation.
4. Meeting the needs of underserved groups.
5. Community participation.

Table 2.1   Focus of targets for 'Health For All' by the year 2000 in Europe

Targets 1–12: Health For All
1. Equity in health
2. Adding years to life
3. Better opportunities for the disabled
4. Reducing disease and disability
5. Eliminating measles, polio, neonatal tetanus, congenital rubella, diphtheria, congenital syphilis and indigenous malaria
6. Increased life expectation at birth
7. Reduced infant mortality
8. Reduced maternal mortality
9. Combating disease of the circulation
10. Combating cancer
11. Reducing accidents
12. Stopping the increase in suicide

Targets 13–17: Life-styles Conducive to Health For All
13. Developing healthy public policies
14. Developing social support systems
15. Improving knowledge and motivation for healthy behaviour
16. Promoting positive health behaviour
17. Decreasing health-damaging behaviour

Targets 18–25: Producing Healthy Environments
18. Policies for healthy environments
19. Monitoring, assessment and control of environmental risks
20. Controlling water pollution
21. Protecting against air pollution
22. Improving food safety
23. Protecting against hazardous wastes
24. Improving housing conditions
25. Protecting against work-related health risks

Targets 26–31: Providing Appropriate Care
26. A health care system based on primary health care
27. Distribution of resources according to need
28. Re-orientating primary medical care
29. Developing teamwork
30. Co-ordinating services
31. Ensuring quality of services

Targets 32–38: Support for Health Development
32. Developing a research base for health for all
33. Implementing policies for health for all
34. Management and delivery of resources
35. Health information systems
36. Training and deployment of staff
37. Education of people in non-health sectors
38. Assessment of health technologies

Health Promotion: A New Concept for the New Public Health

Out of the arguments and discussions generated by the World Health Organization's strategy a new concept has emerged and been developed – the concept of *health promotion*.[30] It is clear from our understanding of the way in which health improved in the past that if we are to achieve the potential for good health which is possible, a broad-based approach will be necessary. From this perspective health promotion as the means to health for all is seen as a process of enabling people to increase control over and improve their health. Health itself is seen as a resource for everyday life, rather than an end in itself.

Principles of Health Promotion

The experience of those active in this field since 1974 has helped to define five principles of health promotion:

1. Health promotion actively involves the population in the setting of every-day life rather than focussing on people who are at risk for specific conditions and in contact with medical services.
2. Health promotion is directed towards action on the causes of ill-health.
3. Health promotion uses many different approaches which combine to improve health. These include education and information, community development and organization, health advocacy and legislation.
4. Health promotion depends particularly on public participation.
5. Health professionals – especially those in primary health care – have an important part to play in nurturing health promotion and enabling it to take place.

At the 1986 Ottawa Conference on Health Promotion, these principles were developed further as the 'Ottawa Charter for Health Promotion.'[31] The Charter stresses in particular the necessity to:

1. *Build public policies which support health.* Health promotion goes beyond health care and makes health an agenda item for policy makers in all areas of governmental and organizational action. Health promotion requires that the obstacles to the adoption of health promoting policies be identified in non-medical sectors together with ways of removing them. The aim must be to make the healthier choices the easier choices.
2. *Create supportive environments.* Health promotion recognizes that both at the global level and at the local level human health is bound up with the way in which we treat nature and the environment. Societies which exploit their environments without attention to ecology, reap the effects of that exploitation in ill-health and social problems. Health cannot be separated from other goals and changing patterns of life. Work and leisure have a definite impact on health. Health promotion, therefore, must create living and

working conditions that are safe, stimulating, satisfying and enjoyable.
3. *Strengthen community action.* Health promotion works through effective community action. At the heart of this process are communities having their own power and having control of their own initiatives and activities. This means that professionals must learn new ways of working with individuals and communities – working for and with rather than on them.
4. *Develop personal skills.* Health promotion supports personal and social development through providing information, education for health and helping people to develop the skills which they need to make healthy choices. By doing so it enables people to exercise more control over their own health and over their environments, making it possible for people to learn throughout life, to prepare themselves for all of its stages and to cope with chronic illness and injuries. This has to be assisted in the school, at home, at work and in community settings.
5. *Reorientate health services.* The responsibility for health promotion in health services is shared among individuals, community groups, health professionals, medical care workers, bureaucracies and governments. They must work together towards a health care system which contributes to the pursuit of health.

The role of the medical sector must develop towards health promotion beyond its responsibility for providing treatment services. To do this it will need to recognize that most of the causes of ill-health lie outside the direct influence of the medical sector and it must be willing to work with those in a position to influence these causes.

Issues raised by Health For All: A Conflict Between Prevention and Treatment?

The debate which surrounds the renaissance of public health is often couched in adversarial terms between prevention and treatment. A conflict of sorts between the two approaches has a long history. In ancient Greece, for the worshippers of Hygieia, health was the natural order of things, a positive attribute to which people were entitled if they governed their lives wisely.[2] According to this view the most important function of medicine was to discover and teach the natural laws which would ensure a healthy mind in a healthy body. More sceptical, the followers of Asclepius believed that the chief role of the physician was to treat disease and to restore health by correcting any imperfections caused by the accidents of birth and life. Quite who should be held responsible for ill-health has long been an item for debate. In the mid-nineteenth century Neumann,[32] arguing for an extended role for the State in public health and the provision of medical care, put it as follows:

The State argues that its responsibility is to protect people's property rights. For most people the only property which they possess is their health; therefore the State has a responsibility to protect people's health.

In general, this point of view, albeit in what we would now see as a paternalistic form, seems to have triumphed and to this day an inscription above the door of the borough public health department in Southwark, South London proclaims 'the Health of the people is the highest law' (Fig. 2.6). However, in recent years, and coinciding with the revival of public health, there has also been a revival of the argument over the responsibility for health with a modern 'victim-blaming' view attracting considerable support in some quarters. The issue is complicated by a widespread move against paternalistic forms of administration and services, as part of a general move towards participative as opposed to representative democracy. In the ensuing confusion it has been possible for some governments to construe that the public no longer wishes to have public services.

The potential danger of a polarization of views between prevention and treatment has been discussed by Professor Morris in a paper entitled 'Are Health Services Important to the Peoples Health?'[33] It is apparent that treatment plays a particularly important part in alleviating the disability of established conditions, particularly in the elderly.

In public health it is customary to divide prevention into three types: primary, secondary and tertiary. Primary prevention together with health promotion has as its aim the prevention of disorders before they occur, either by positive strategies to affect those factors conducive to disorders in an entire, defined population or else in a subgroup of that population who are identified as being at risk.

Such strategies are only possible when causes are known and preventive strategies are feasible. When they are not it is necessary to fall back on secondary prevention, involving early diagnosis and treatment, including screening programmes, with the aim of limiting the course of an illness and reducing the risk of recurrence.

When even that is not possible recourse must be had to tertiary prevention aimed at reducing the burden of disability to the individual and to society and obtaining optimal health under the circumstances. Clearly, with an ageing population and in our current state of knowledge, there is a host of chronic conditions that we do not know how to prevent but where treatment may make all the difference to the quality of life and thus to health. To the extent to which death is itself inevitable sometime, high-quality terminal care is a form of tertiary prevention.

Examples of chronic conditions where modern treatments can effect dramatic improvements in the quality of life include the effectiveness of hip – and lens – replacement operations and the removal of the prostate gland. It is likely that there will be many advances in this category in the coming years.

The common theme of all public health strategies of health promotion and prevention is a shift in the direction of health of the entire population, rather than a concern solely with individuals.

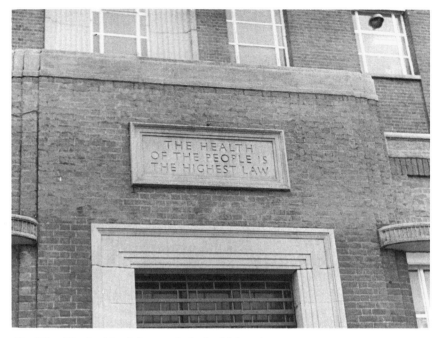

Fig. 2.6.   The health of the people is the highest law.

This text was originally taken from Cicero De-Legibus Book 3, 3, 8. Contained in Benhams Book of Quotations, 1948.

These principles are illustrated by reference to hypertension and stroke as public health problems.[34–38] Between 15 and 20 per cent of adults have raised blood pressure, the existence of which is most important for the development of heart disease and stroke, as well as for conditions of the kidneys and eyes. Often it causes no symptoms until it has been present for a long time and many people are unaware of their condition. It is, however, only one of several risk factors for heart disease and stroke; other factors include cigarette smoking, raised blood cholesterol levels, diabetes and obesity. A comprehensive approach to the problem of hypertension would include:

1. Health promotion and primary prevention: to remove the risk factors from the population through changes in behaviour and life-style, supported by appropriate public policies and health education.
2. Secondary prevention: screening of at-risk groups for hypertension backed up by counselling, health education and treatment where appropriate.
3. Tertiary prevention: rehabilitation, treatment, counselling and education for stroke victims and those with hypertensive heart disease.

Control of high blood pressure once it has been identified requires people to adhere strictly to certain measures throughout their lifetime. These may

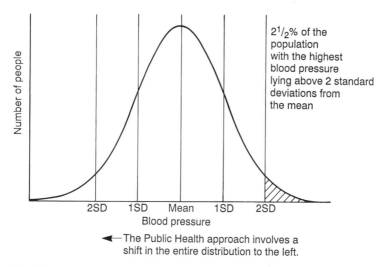

Fig. 2.7.   The normal distribution of blood pressure in a human population.

include changes in exercise, diet and the management of stress with or without prescribed medicine. At present it seems that blood pressure control can be described according to the rule of halves:

- half of hypertensives are known,
- half of known hypertensives are being treated, and
- half of those hypertensives who are being treated are being effectively treated.

As a result, many avoidable deaths from heart disease and stroke occur annually, strokes alone accounting for between 5 and 10 per cent of years of life lost before age 75 in developed countries.

The distinction between a conventional clinical approach to the problem and a public health approach is illustrated in Fig. 2.7. Many biological dimensions can be described statistically by a normal distribution curve (Gaussian curve) which divides the population up into segments or standard deviations from the population mean. Two standard deviations above and below the mean includes 95 per cent of the population. In the case of hypertension those people with a diastolic blood pressure greater than 105 mmHg constitute the 2.5 per cent of the population most at risk of heart disease and stroke. The conventional medical approach is to try to identify these people and modify their blood pressure by changes in life-style with or without pharmacological treatment. However, from a public health perspective, although members of this group are individually at greatest risk, collectively they do not make the greatest contribution to the numbers of heart disease and stroke victims. They are to be found in the numerically much larger second category of risk lying between one and two standard deviations from the mean. The alternative of identifying and treating this large proportion of the population is ethically unacceptable.

It follows from this that a public health approach to the problem of hypertension involves achieving a shift to the left of the complete population distribution through general measures to reduce risk factors among the entire population, none of whom individually may ever know whether they would have developed problems had they not adopted the proposed changes. Clearly the kind of changes which are indicated in relation to exercise, nutrition alcohol and tobacco consumption are not totally dependent on individual choice but are influenced by prevailing economic, legislative and social policies as well as the prevailing cultural milieu. The lessons to be drawn from this specific case are applicable to many other contemporary public health issues.

The Need for Comprehensive Strategies of Health Promotion

The need for a broad view which integrates preventive and treatment medicine and acknowledges the wider political and social dimensions of health is not new. In 1941 the medical historian Sigerist[39] noted that any national health programme ought to include:

1. Free education including health education.
2. The best possible working and living conditions.
3. The best possible means of rest and recreation.
4. A system of health institutions and medical personnel available to all responsible for the population's health, ready and able to advise and help them in the maintenance of health and in its restoration when prevention broke down.
5. Centres of medical training and research.

The need was made explicit in the United Kingdom in the Beveridge report of 1942, which to a large extent represented a consensus brought about by the appalling effects of the recession in the 1930s. The plan was put forward as part of an attack upon the 'five giant evils':

> the physical *Want* with which it is directly concerned, upon *Disease* which ofen causes Want and brings many other troubles in its train, upon *Ignorance* which no democracy can afford among its citizens, upon *Squalor* which arises mainly through the haphazard distribution of industry and population and upon *Idleness* which destroys wealth and corrupts people whether they are well fed or not, when they are idle.

Although the paternalism of the institutions which developed from Beveridge may be unacceptable to a new generation, this analysis makes quite clear the political nature of health problems and particularly of primary prevention. They confirm the view of Virchow that 'Medicine is a Social Science and politics is nothing else but medicine on a large scale'.[41] Clearly an interest in health must be a legitimate concern of all members of the community and not solely of doctors and health workers.

Ever since the inception of the British National Health Services (NHS) only a very small proportion of funds has been given over to the promotion of good health and the prevention of disease. In 1976 the Department of Health published *Prevention and Health: Everybody's Business*, which was intended to stimulate discussion about the scope for modern preventive medicine.[25] This was followed up by the DHSS report *Priorities for Health and Personal Social Services in England* (1976) and *The Way Forward* (1977).[42,43] The Royal Commission on the NHS, reporting in 1979, concluded that a 'significant improvement in the health of all people of the U.K. can come through prevention'.[44] The members of the commission 'considered that there were major areas where government action could produce rapid and certain results: a much tougher attitude towards smoking, towards preventing road accidents and mitigating their results, a clear commitment to fluoridation and a programme to combat alcoholism' were specifically mentioned but they also considered that such action had to be matched by other measures:

> We saw a need for more emphasis on health education and the develop-
> ment and monitoring of its techniques, far greater involvement of GPs
> and other health professionals and far better in-service training for
> teachers in health education. The imaginative use of radio and television
> would be important. We felt that much more could be done to emphasise
> the positive virtues of health and the risks of an unhealthy lifestyle and
> that this should include environmental and occupational hazards as well
> as personal behaviour. We were concerned that Local Authorities should
> not let standards of environmental health slip. We considered that the
> N.H.S. needed to face its responsibilities for prevention.

In coming to their recommendations, the Black working party identified three objectives:

1. To give children a better start in life.
2. To encourage good health among a greater proportion of the population by preventive and educational action.
3. To reduce the risks of premature death for disabled people and to improve the quality of life whether in the community or in the institutions and as far as possible reduce the need for the latter.

The group discussed their recommendations in terms of action within the health services and action in other policy areas with a particular emphasis on the need to abolish childhood poverty and to tackle on a multidisciplinary front the toll of death and disability caused by domestic and road traffic accidents.

More recently, the British Government has accepted the need to take active steps to develop primary medical care and has conducted a fundamental review of the Public Health Function in the light of failures of infectious disease control and environmental health monitoring and weakness in the relationship between the medical and other sectors of relevant public policy.[45–47] In

Canada, in keeping with its vanguard position, the government has embraced the HFA 2000 Strategy as part of its own commitment to a defined health promotion strategy.[46–48]

Reorientating Primary Care

The reorientation of medical care towards health promotion, prevention and primary medical care is an essential part of the World Health Organization Strategy.[28,49,50] This reorientation involves a further shift from primary medical care (a medical concept based on the equitable availability and accessibility of good quality preventive and treatment services from a team of health workers based in the community) to primary health care, which is a social concept going much wider in that it is concerned with populations as well as individuals and that it seeks to involve a range of people other than trained health workers. The implications for training and organization in achieving this paradigm shift are considerable, particularly in respect of the need to achieve real public participation and intersectoral working.

The World Health Organization concept of primary health care incorporates a recognition that health care should be planned to relate to the resources available. It sees primary health care as the most local part of a comprehensive health system and it recognizes that the public should participate both individually and collectively in the planning and implementation of health care.

The Peckham Pioneer Health Centre as a Model of Primary Health Care

Primary health care as envisaged by WHO is hard to find. One celebrated example was the Peckham Pioneer Health Centre established in South London in the 1930s. The initial idea of the Peckham Centre arose from the meeting of two people: the late Dr G. Scott Williamson and his colleague Dr Innes Pearse, later to be his wife. Williamson was a pathologist who had become fascinated by the lack of susceptibility to disease which accompanies health and which is different from acquired immunity.[51,52] He sought conditions in which health was to be found and could be encouraged and studied, and this led to the idea of the health centre. On the other hand, Pearse's experience in the early 1920s was in one of the earliest Infant Welfare Clinics in a working-class district, where she gained the conviction that advice on the control of conception should be given in the context of the family as a whole.

The health centre, which emerged in 1935 from the ideas and work of these pioneers and others who became involved, was and remains a remarkable building, consisting of three large concrete platforms one above the other with cantilever supports surrounding a large rectangular central space occupied by a swimming pool on the first floor (Fig. 2.8). The outer walls and those of the swimming pool were of glass, while the front of the building contained a series of bow windows with sections which could fold back to form open balconies; the building featured partition walls between rooms allowing flexibility in the use of the floor area.

On the second floor there were private consulting rooms, reception rooms, changing rooms, a small laboratory and rooms for craftwork and meetings. At

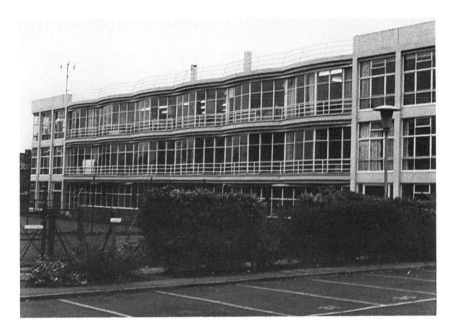

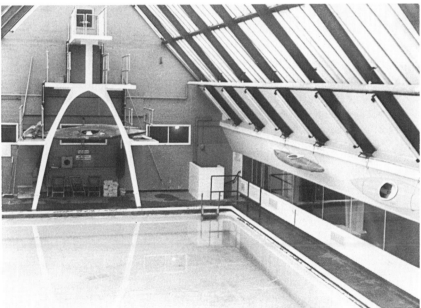

Fig. 2.8.   The Peckham Pioneer Health Centre.

one end of the swimming pool was a gymnasium and at the other a theatre
which could be used for badminton. The swimming pool was overlooked on
one side by a self-service cafeteria and on the other by a recreation room used

for dancing. The ground floor contained a day nursery with room for an infant dormitory.

In planning the new centre it was felt that the population should be essentially healthy and that it should include a cross-section by age. It would be for people to come to the centre rather than for the centre to proselytize, and what happened in the centre would be for the members to decide. It would be continuously available in leisure time and its aim was to provide opportunities whenever an opportunity could be taken up – a reflection of the strong belief in Montessori theories.

The scientists themselves were to become one of the groups forming part of the cultural diversity of the centre, and their task was to observe the actions of the individual and the family – and their interactions – as well as carrying out physiological studies of each individual and each family. The knowledge collected by the scientists was then to be returned to each family for their own use.

The initial equipment consisted of a few books in the library, a billiard table, games for the children and a piano. The intention was that the family members would acquire and furnish the equipment they wanted for themselves. The pioneers saw the centre as a building to be furnished with people and with their actions, and they achieved a design which invited social contact. It was to be a comfortable place providing a focus of the sort provided in former times by the village hall and green.

In keeping with the philosophy of the centre as a community resource any family within one mile of the centre could join. This was regarded as 'pram walking distance'. There was to be a family subscription of one shilling per week which brought with it responsibilities and privileges of membership, viz.:

1. A periodic health overhaul for each individual of a member family.
2. The use of the centre and its equipment. This was to be free to all children of school age belonging to a member family, though adults were to pay a small additional sum for each activity (Table 2.2).

The community aspect of the centre was underwritten by principles which are probably fundamental in the pursuit of health:

1. There was no organizer. It was for the members to organize and choose for themselves how the building would be used. There was an emphasis throughout on self-determination which was symbolized by the self-service cafeteria, a method of organization arrived at by choice rather than expediency.
2. Emphasis was on ordinary achievement. Experts were not allowed to dominate any activity by taking it over. This created an atmosphere where everybody felt able to try activities, and not be afraid of failing or being mediocre, e.g. swimming.

From its opening in 1935 until the advent of the Second World War, the Peckham Experiment continued to develop with increasing numbers of family members and a growing sense of identity and loyalty. The building was evacuated at the beginning of the war at the request of the police and was later

Table 2.2   The Facilities at Peckham Health Centre

Welfare and Educational
Antenatal clinic; postnatal clinic; birth control clinic; infant welfare clinic, care of the toddler; nursery school; immunization service; schoolchildren's medical examinations; vocational guidance; sex instruction for adolescents; girls' and boys' clubs; youth centres; sports clubs and recreation clubs of all sorts; keep fit and gymnastic classes; adult cultural education; music, debates, drama, any event desired by members; citizens advice bureau; holiday organizations; outings and expeditions; the bar; billiards; dancing; social gatherings.

Therapeutic
Marriage advice bureau; mothers' clinic; child guidance clinic; poor man's lawyer; social worker; hospital follow-up overhaul; rehabilitation clinic.

used as a munitions factory. Twenty nine young families with 50 children under 5 years of age went to live at a farm in Bromley which had been acquired by the Peckham Centre and which was wanted by its members to provide fresh food and milk. However, the country experiment apparently failed for financial reasons after about a year.

In 1945, as a result principally of the demand by former members of the centre, the building was reopened, and of the 875 families who were members at the beginning of the war, 550 families immediately rejoined. Over the next 3 years, however, the financial support available to maintain the building proved inadequate and in 1951 the pioneers were compelled to sell the building to the local authority.

Ironically, support for the centre was not forthcoming from the National Health Service, apparently because the ethic was not compatible with the ascendant values of the therapeutic era. Subsequently, the use of the Peckham building has changed and while maintaining links with the original ideas bears little resemblance to the integrated ecological focus of its originators. The medical facilities are now used as a diagnostic service by South London family doctors and the main part of the building has become the Frobisher Adult Education Centre, with a large catchment area and a director.

At the present time, within many countries there is an excitement and energy attached to preventive medicine and primary medical care which was not there 20 years ago. Some countries have passed special legislation to assist the shift in emphasis from hospital- to community-based services; several have produced 'National Health for All Strategies' and, perhaps most encouragingly, there is a great deal of interest and activity in developing health promotion, preventive medicine and primary care at the local level. In some countries medical students now actively opt for careers outside hospitals. Yet in England and Wales, for example, where many of the desirable elements for the development of primary health care exist, considerable problems remain, not least in the inner-city areas of the conurbations and on the peripheral public housing estates (Table 2.3).[44] In these areas the gap between the health experience of different social classes has continued to increase. Concern about

Table 2.3 Elements of a good system of primary health care in the United Kingdom

---

1. Existence and development of family medicine
2. Existence of a professional body to develop standards (Royal College of General Practitioners)
3. Training programmes for primary health care staff
4. Specified training requirements
5. Postgraduate co-ordinators (General Practice Deans)
6. Postgraduate training centres
7. A health centre building programme
8. A team approach
9. Influence of psychodynamic and social science knowledge on medical practice
10. Availability of a population denominator for primary care (the list of registered patients)
11. Small group meetings for medical staff
12. Consumer representation (Community Health Councils)
13. Preventive medicine and health promotion initiatives

---

the standards of services in these areas has led to a number of studies and reports.[45,53-56]

In part the problem seems to lie with the extent to which some or all of these elements exist and are appropriately developed; this is highly variable, especially within the inner areas of some of the cities. In particular, there is a general lack of what might be called the epidemiological or population view of primary health care as espoused by Tudor Hart and Kark, and there is a great need for the injection of epidemiological skills into the normal functioning of primary health care teams.[57,58] The development of appropriate information systems based on the age-sex register, probably supplemented by intermittent sample surveys of the practice population to assess risk factors and answer specific questions, will be a necessary step in providing the conceptual framework for a rational and comprehensive approach to preventive medicine and health promotion. Such developments in information could provide much needed planning information to Local and District Health Authorities and are becoming increasingly feasible with the advent of microcomputerts.[59,60]

Concern about the inner cities needs to be set against the positive initiatives which have been taken, particularly in relation to the activities of the members of the Royal College of General Practitioners. A series of reports has identified specific areas where advances can be made in health promotion and preventive medicine based on general practice, and the growing interest in the quality of care is reflected in the publication of a recent consultation document.[61,67]

These very positive initiatives from the royal College of General Practitioners have led to an assumption by some, that in future preventive medicine will be organized and provided by primary medical care teams centred on general practice. One consequence of this has been that the community health services which have traditionally been responsible for ensuring population coverage of preventive measures are in a state of uncertainty as to their future. On the face of it, it seems desirable to run down services which in many ways both parallel those provided by general practitioners and, in addition, suffer from the weaknesses attributed to vertical programmes.[68] However, despite the positive trends and initiatives in British general practice already described, there is little to indicate that doctors as prime movers are ready for primary health as opposed to primary medical care.

A recent survey in one British health region underlined the fact that whereas some progressive practitioners are keen to develop participative styles and intersectoral working most are still tightly locked into a medical model. Of 120 general practices in Birmingham which took part in the survey, whereas immunization was available in 92 per cent, family planning in 85 per cent and antenatal care in 78 per cent, mother and baby clinics were available in only 49 per cent, developmental screening in 37 per cent and parentcraft classes in 20 per cent; only 2 per cent of practices offered self-help groups and 54 per cent of general practitioners thought that they did not have the time to do preventive work.[69] As the 120 completed questionnaires represented a response rate of only 35 per cent, all of these figures are likely to be over-estimates, lending support to the notion that those who foresee the imminent takeover of the public health function by medically orientated general practitioners are suffering from the fantasy that what is exceptional is in fact normative. When it comes to the kind of community-development linkage with primary health care which is to be found in non-industrial countries and which should be regarded as just as important in, for example, inner-city areas of the United Kingdom, there is nothing to suggest that general practitioners regard this kind of work as having anything to do with them. Taken together with the generally negative response from doctors to the recent suggestions by the Cumberlege Report that primary care should be organized on a geographical basis, it seems likely that parallel and indeed vertical and selective programmes will exist in primary care for the foreseeable future.[70]

Community Participation and Intersectoral Action

The elements of the Ottawa Charter, which focus on the creation of environments which are supportive to health and on the enabling of communities through the development of personal skills and health advocacy, are in a real sense a challenge to professional practice as it is found throughout the World.[31,71] Professional power and prestige is contingent upon the acquisition of specific knowledge and skills which are exchanged for money in return for a service; the autonomy of the professional in the market is central as is his or her freedom to refuse a client. There is no commitment either to population coverage or to sharing power and demystifying knowledge. In this sense, there is a real conflict between the clinical model based on individual transactions and the public health model based on a social contract with entire communities. The consequence of this is that there is a great deal of rhetoric about public participation but a marked unwillingness to really engage in the processes which would bring it about. Most professionals and welfare bureaucracies function only on the lower half of Arnstein's ladder of citizen participation:[72]

Citizen control
Delegated power
Partnership
Placation
Consultation
Informing
Therapy
Manipulation

Yet in wishing for people to take increased responsibility for their own health it is necessary to recognize the close relationship between risk-taking behaviour and lack of empowerment.[73]

References

1. Kickbusch, I. (1986). Health promotion strategies for action. *Canadian Journal of Public Health* **77** (5), 321–6.
2. McKeown, T. (1976). *The role of Medicine – Dream, Mirage or Nemesis*. Nuffield Provincial Hospitals Trust, London.
3. Kaye, T. (1829). *The Stranger in Liverpool*. T. Kaye, Liverpool.
4. Chave, S.P.W. (1984). Duncan of Liverpool – and some lessons for today. *Community Medicine* **6**, 61–71.
5. Kearns, G. (1986). Private property and public health reform in England 1830–70. *Soc. Sci. Med.* **26** (1), 187–99.
6. Cartwright, F.F. (1977). *A Social History of Medicine*. Longmans, London.
7. Fraser, W.M. (1947). *Duncan of Liverpool*. Hamish Hamilton, London.
8. Hardy, G. (1981). *William Rathbone and the Early History of District Nursing*. G.W. and A. Hesketh, Ormskirk.
9. Lane, T. (1986). *Liverpool – Gateway of Empire*. Lawrence and Wishart, London.
10. Ashton, J.R. (1979). Poverty and health in Britain today. *Public Health* **93**, 89–94.
11. Godber, G.E. (1986). Medical officers of health and health services. *Community Medicine* **8** (1), 1–14.
12. Townsend, P. and Davidson, N. (1980). *Inequalities in Health – The Black Report*. Penguin, Harmondsworth.
13. Whitehead, M. (1987). *The Health Divide – Inequalities in Health*. Health Education Council, London.
14. Smith, F.B., Francis, Barrymore (1979). *The Peoples Health*. Croom Helm, London.
15. Illich, I. (1975). *Medical Nemesis – The Expropriation of Health*. Marion Boyars,
16. Boston Women's Health Book Collective (1984). *The New Our Bodies Ourselves*. Simon and Schuster, New York.
17. Levin, L.S., Katz, A.H. and Holst, E. (1977). *Self-care*. Croom Helm, London.
18. WHO Europe (1983). *Self-help and Health in Europe*. WHO, Geneva.
19. Lalonde, M. (1974). *A New Perspective on the Health of Canadians*. Minister of Supply and Services.
20. Doyal, L. (1981). *The Political Economy of Health*. Pluto Press, London.
21. Navarro, V. (1976). *Medicine Under Capitalism*. Croom Helm, London.
22. Milio, N. (1986). *Promoting Health Through Public Policy*, Canadian Public Health Association. Ottawa, Canada.
23. St. George, D. and Draper, P. (1981). A health policy for Europe. *Lancet* **ii**, 463–5.

24. Department of Health Education and Welfare (1979). *Healthy People*. The Surgeon General's report on Health Promotion and Disease Prevention. DHEW Publications, Washington, D.C.

25. HMSO (1976). *Prevention and Health: Everybody's Business*. A reassessment of Public and Personal Health. HMSO, London.

26. World Health Organization (1981). *Global Strategy for Health For All by the Year 2000*. WHO, Geneva.

27. World Health Organization (1978). *Alma Ata 1977. Primary Health Care*. WHO, UNICEF, Geneva.

28. WHO Europe. (1981). *Regional Strategy for Attaining Health For All by the Year 2000*. EUR/RC 3018. rev 1. WHO, Copenhagen.

29. WHO Europe (1985). *Targets for Health For All*. WHO, Copenhagen.

30. WHO Europe (1984). *Health Promotion*. A discussion document on the concepts and principles. WHO, Copenhagen.

31. World Health Organization, Health and Welfare Canada, Canadian Public Health Association (1986). *Ottawa Charter for Health Promotion*. WHO, Copenhagen.

32. Neumann, S. (1847). *Die Offentliches Gesundeheitstflege und das eigenthum*. Berlin. Quoted in H. Sigerist *op. cit.*

33. Morris, J.N. (1980). Are health services important to the people's health? *British Medical Journal* **280**, 167–8.

34. Tudor-Hart, J. (1980). *Hypertension*. Churchill Livingstone, Edinburgh.

35. Rose, G. (1981). Strategy of prevention: lessons from cardiovascular disease. *British Medical Journal* **282**, 1847.

36. Rose, G. (1985). Sick individuals and sick populations. *International Journal of Epidemiology* **14**, 32–8.

37. Rose, G. (1985). The strategy of cardiovascular disease control. *Health and Hygiene* **6**, 105–108.

38. World Health Organization (1982). *Prevention of Coronary Heart Disease*. Technical Report Series 678. WHO, Geneva.

39. Sigerist, H. (1941). *Medicine and Human Welfare*. Oxford University Press, Oxford.

40. Beveridge, Sir W. (1942). *Social Insurance and Allied Services*. Cmd. 6404, 6405. HMSO, London.

41. Virchow, R.L.K. (1848). *Die Medizinische Reform*, p. 2. Quoted in Sigerist, H.E. (1941). *Medicine and Human Welfare*, p. 93. Yale University Press, New Haven.

42. Department of Health and Social Security (1976). *Priorities for Health and Social Service in England*. HMSO, London.

43. Department of Health and Social Security (1977). *The Way Forward – Priorities in the Health and Social Services*. HMSO, London.

44. Merrison, A. (1979). *Royal Commission on the National Health Service*, HMSO, London.

45. Department of Health and Social Security (1987). *Promoting Better Health – The Government Programme for Improving Primary Health Care*. Cmnd. 249. HMSO, London.

46. Acheson, E.D. (1988). *On the State of the Public Health*. The Fourth Duncan Lecture. *Public Health* **102**, 431–37.

47. The Acheson Report (1988). *Public Health in England*. The Report of the Committee of Enquiry into the future development of the Public Health Function. Cmnd. 289. HMSO, London.

48. Epp, J. (1986). Achieving health for all: A framework for health promotion. *Canadian Journal of Public Health* **77** (6), 393–424.

49. Vuori, H. (1981). Primary health care in industrialized countries. In Die Allgemeinpraxix: Das Zentrum der Artzlichen, Grundverorgung Gottleib Duttwierer – Institut Ruschlikon, Zurich, pp. 83–111.

50. Hellberg, H. (1987). Health for all and primary health care in Europe. *Public Health* **101**, 151–7.
51. Ashton, J. (1977). The Peckham Pioneer Health Centre: A reappraisal. *Community Health* **8**, 132–7.
52. Pearse, I.H. and Crocker, L.H. (1943). *The Peckham Experiment*. Allen and Unwin, London.
53. Harding, W.G. (1981). *The Primary Health Care Team*. Report of a Joint Working Party of the Standing Advisory Committee and the Standing Nursing and Midwifery Advisory Committee. HMSO, London.
54. Acheson, E.D. (1981). *Primary Health Care in Inner London*. Report of a Study Group. Commissioned by the London Health Planning Consortium, HMSO, London.
55. Jarman, B. (1981). *A Survey of Primary Care in London*. Report prepared for the Royal College of General Practitioners, London.
56. Bolden, K.J. (1981). *Inner City*. Occasional Paper 19. Royal College of General Practitioners, London.
57. Tudor Hart, J. (1981). 'A new kind of doctor', *Journal of the Royal Society of Medicine*. **74**, 871–83.
58. Kark, S.L. (1981). *The Practice of Community Orientated Primary Health Care*. Appleton, Century, Crofts, New York.
59. Ashton, J.R. (1983). Micro-computers for general practitioners – an opportunity for collaboration. *Journal of the Royal College of General Practitioners*. **33**, 455–6.
60. Horder, R.J. (1983). Practice observed – General practice in 2000. Alma Ata Declaration. *British Medical Journal* **286** 191–4.
61. Royal College of General Practitioners (1981). Health and Prevention in Primary Care. Report from *General Practice* **19**.
62. Royal College of General Practitioners (1981). Prevention of Arterial Disease in General Practice. Report from *General Practice* **19**.
63. Royal College of General Practitioners (1981). Prevention of Psychiatric Disorders in General Practice. Report from *General Practice* **20**.
64. Royal College of General Practitioners (1981). Family Planning, an Exercise in Preventive Medicine. Report from *General Practice* **21**.
65. Royal College of General Practitioners (1981). Healthier Children – Thinking Prevention. Report from *General Practice* **22**.
66. Royal College of General Practitioners (1983). *Promoting Prevention. Occasional Paper 22*, Royal College of General Practitioners, London.
67. Royal College of General Practitioners (1985). *Towards Quality in General Practice*. A Council Consultation Document. Royal College of General Practitioners, London.
68. Rifkin, S.B. and Walt, G. (1986). Why health improves: Defining the issues concerning 'primary health care' and 'selective primary health care'. *Soc. Sci. Med.* **23** (6), 559–66.
69. Hamlin, M. (1984). *Children and Prevention in General Practice*. Department of Psychology, North Birmingham Health Authority, Birmingham.
70. HMSO (1986). *Neighbourhood Nursing – A Focus for Care*. Report of the Community Nursing Review. HMSO, London.
71. Chambers, R. (1983). *Rural Development – Putting the Last First*. Longmans, London.
72. Arnstein, S. (1969). 'A ladder of public participation'. *Journal of the American Institute of Planners*. Quoted in N. Wates and C. Knevitt, (1987) *Community Architecture*, Penguin Books, London.
73. Ashton, J. (1983). Risk assessment. *British Medical Journal* **286**, 1843.

3   The Change Makers

What is Health?

The question 'What is health and thereby health promotion?' continues to de-energize all those involved in this activity. Debates about the meaning of health have led to more conflict and inaction than they have solved. To clear a way through this morass, let us state quite clearly that health promotion is an activity whose basis resides in gaining change, change to promote health. The methods of change are its subject. It draws on the skills and practice of change that are found well-established in politics, economics, the media, therapy, education, advocacy, legislation etc.

The object of health promotion is the promotion of health. To shift a gear and move away from this inward-looking tautology we must take a pragmatic and commonsense approach to the meaning of health, an approach which asserts that health is gained and lost in the real world in almost every action we indulge in: in our work, at our leisure, with our family and friends. It is easy to recognize that all of these contribute to our health, to our being able to live socially and economically fulfilling lives.

Health promotion as an activity is distinguished from its predecessors, health education and community medicine, by two features. First, it recognizes the proposition that health is bigger than the prevention of disease, illness and disability. It is, therefore, inclusive and its rhetoric includes ideas of participation, multisectorality, populisms, etc. It is interested in big systems – in the body politic, in education (not just health education, but general education through life, which is probably a better indicator of health and well-being than investment in medical care) and in a thriving economy. Secondly, while recognizing the important contribution that individuals can make to their own health it concentrates on mass effects and the creation of environments, and options which encourage healthy choices.

The accent of health promotion is on change: change as a society as well as at an individual and an organizational level. Because of this direction, one of the primary interests of the health promotion enthusiast or practitioner must be on the changes which are occurring in our society, the *trends*.

Why Trends?

Trends are important because the health promoter – the 'change maker' – needs to recognize and use the changes that are constant in our society. The movement of people from the land to cities in newly industrializing societies, the movement of people away from cities into the countryside in the so-called post-industrial phase, and the probable movement back to the cities to gentrify architecturally rich, but decaying, inner cities, are all examples of change – change that has occurred, or seems likely to occur. Changes like this can be seen as a movement in a stream and are called trends.

Living in today's society can be seen as a multitude of unconnected events. We move from one event to another, rarely pausing to notice any pattern or structure. However, the patterns are there and they are the basic data for the commentator on human events, the social scientist or the historian.

To the change maker the importance of trends cannot be neglected. The major trends of today will collectively shape our future. They are powerful phenomena so why should health promoters battle in their own small way to introduce change when their objectives may at any moment be hit with enormous force by a major trend, or smashed into obscurity? – 'Oh I remember that, it was one of those fads the health people tried to get us to do!'

Trends From The People

One skill of the 'change makers' can probably be defined as the riding of the waves, a kind of social science surfing. This skill involves recognizing a trend (a ripple of change which is starting to occur), moving with it, learning about it while it develops into a wave, and then riding it and attempting to steer a course.

Trend recognition

John Naisbett[1], a professional commentator on the future, has said that the most reliable way to anticipate the future is by understanding the present.

Naisbett's methodology is based on content analysis. The roots of this approach are to be found in the Second World War. To gain some idea of the state of German public opinion, US scientists began to analyse the content of German local newspapers. By carefully logging stories about factory openings and closures, production targets, train arrivals and departures, lists of dead and wounded, they could work out what was happening and what were the trends.

Naisbett's organization has applied the same technique to newspapers in the USA. The validity of this approach in predicting trends is based on the experience that, for economic reasons, there is a constant and finite amount of space in newspapers. So when something new is introduced, something else or a combination of things must be omitted. Because the choice of items is constrained by space, for societies to add new preoccupations, they must drop old ones. Concern in the 1960s about racism was to some extent displaced in the 1970s by feminism and environmental issues and, in the 1980s, ageing and the grey revolution have become major issues. Societies, as represented by newspapers, seem oddly human – people can only keep so many concerns or problems in their heads at any one time, adding new ones means refocussing old ones.

Naisbett's method is also free of the bias of prediction and opinion because only real events are recorded and totalled. The trends of the future are shaped by the events of the present.

Naisbetts's Megatrends

Using content analysis of the local press in the USA and a number of other sources, Naisbett, in his book *Megatrends*, suggests that there are 10 major transformations taking place *in the USA*.[1] These transformations are as follows:

1. *Industrial to information society.* Although Americans continue to think that they live in an industrial society, they have, in fact, changed to an economy based on the creation and distribution of information.
2. *High technology, high touch.* They are moving in the dual directions of high tech/high touch, matching each new technology with a compensatory human response and contact.
3. *From national to global economy.* The USA no longer has the luxury of operating within an isolated, self-sufficient, national economic system; it is now part of the global economy. The trend is away from assuming that the USA is and must remain the world's industrial leader as it moves on to other tasks. At the same time, there is a renewed interest in local power and control. The implication is that there is a need to think global and also act local.
4. *Short-term to long-term.* There is a restructuring from a society run by short-term considerations and rewards in favour of dealing with things in much longer time frames.
5. *Centralization and decentralization.* In cities and states, in small organizations and subdivisions, the ability to act innovatively and to achieve results from the bottom up is being rediscovered.
6. *Institutional help to self-help.* There is a movement away from institutional help to more self-help, -care and -control.
7. *Representation to participation.* They are discovering, however slowly, that

the framework of representative democracy is becoming obsolete in an era
of instantaneously shared information.
8. *Hierarchy to network.* They are giving up their dependence on hierarchical
   structures in favour of informal networks.
9. *North to south.* People are moving out of the old northern industrial area to
   the 'sun rise' areas of the south and west.
10. *Either/or to multiple option.* There is a trend away from a narrow either/or
    society with a limited range of personal choices to a 'free-wheeling'
    multiple option society.

Megatrends was first published in the USA in 1984. The trends described are
of that time and for the USA. However, many of the trends described still fit
with uncanny ease in 1988. The information/service-based economy, the
decline of northern industrial cities, the movement south, the rise of self-help,
the development of networks and increasing global communications are all
watchwords of today. Some of the trends are less easy to recognize in
'Thatcher's Britain', e.g. decentralization seems to be giving way to centralization. This probably highlights one of Naisbett's strictures, i.e. trends do
not go in straight lines. It may be, of course, that to gain decentralization in a
country burdened with enormous hierarchical bureaucracies, maintenance
organizations have a built-in tendency to kill innovation and operate according to the rule that centralization is the chosen path to a 'bottom up' approach.
Only time will tell whether power, once it has been drawn to the centre, can be
given away. (Our own feelings are that this will happen but not without
resistance; however, it is easier to overcome a few than to deal with impersonal
bureaucracy.) The centralization/decentralization issue provides a good example to the change maker. Riding the wave, the trend of devolution to the
local level using the rhetoric of decentralization (particularly in the health
service, education and nationalized industry), the British Government in the
1980s has managed, with apparent ease, to ride on a trend and a steer a course
in their chosen direction, i.e. centralization.

Demographic changes in society are also called trends but, in many
respects, they are very different from megatrends. They provide the infrastructure against which the megatrends occur.

Given the proposition that major trends have implications for, and are the
substance of, health promotion, what are the implications? First of all we need
to be sensitive to popular trends and new directions in technology, social
organization and political philosophy. In the short term, we will need to operate
as social entrepreneurs. Keeping in touch with trends is very similar in some
respects to the activity of the business entrepreneur – by defining new products
and markets, people will buy what they want, and people will define the ways in
which they want to gain and keep their health. This is not just social marketing,
taking a predefined health promotion objective and seeing how it can best be
sold to different client segments of the market. The approach involves knowing
that there are many ways to gain health, and then working with the public to
define a wide range of interventions which fit with growing popular concerns.

A social entrepreneur must maintain good grass-root contacts, while at the same time having an eye for the trends that are developing and planning activities/interventions accordingly; very much more of an art than a science, although John Naisbett has shown that scientific/quantitative tools can help.

Megatrends and Health Promotion

Two examples serve to illustrate how trends can both effect and be used by health promotion.

THE GREYING OF AMERICA

One major trend which was not included in the list of megatrends is based on demography. Major changes in the age/sex structure of society are different from the trends in social and technological organization described so far. They are the powerful background against which the megatrends operate. The UK and the USA and many other developed countries are ageing. It used to be said that people did not age – *they died*. Two articles in a major US magazine[2,3] have outlined the changes – personal, demographic, health and social – as the USA ages. Today, many Americans could well live into their 90s. Fastest growing of all is the group aged 85 and over. By 1995, the population of the average US town will look like Florida's population today.

The implications for health promotion in the future are likely to be dramatic. The most obvious and straightforward prediction is an increasing burden on social security and health care. In the next century, when the baby boomers reach old age, the social costs look alarming. The $50 billion spent on health care for the old when President Reagan came into office is expected to reach 200 billion by the year 2000. Between 1980 and 2040, experts project a 160 per cent increase in physician visits by the elderly, a 200 per cent increase in 'days in' hospital care, and a 280 per cent growth in the number of nursing home residents. Between 1988 and 2000, a new 220-bed nursing home will have to be opened every day just to keep the pace with demand. Without a change in the system, pension and health care costs in the USA will account for more than 60 per cent of the federal budget by 2040. Even if we leave aside the question of who is going to pay for America to grow old, the future looks bleak. But is this the case? There are a number of other factors that we should take into account.

The first and most important question to ask is whether the future cohorts of the old are going to be the same as those of the past? If we look at the diseases that are most responsible for disability in older people, we find that a decline into disabling illness and decrepitude is not automatic or necessary. How long or how well one lives depends, in part, on heredity. However, many of the fears people have about ageing are greatly exaggerated. Senility is greatly feared and yet only 15 per cent of those over 65 years suffer serious mental impairment. About half of this is due to Alzheimer's disease, much of the rest is due to heart disease, liver or thyroid trouble, dietary deficiency and *over-medication*, all of which, apart from Alzheimer's disease, is either reversible or entirely preventable.

Sex is important to our identity and well-being, loss of libido and impotence need not be linked to age. The dampening of sexual urges in women, post-menopause, is often related to physical causes such as hot flushes and vaginal dryness which may be alleviated by oestrogen therapy. Older men routinely accept impotence as normal, but it is often due to psychological problems, diabetes, heart disease and chronic alcohol abuse, all again preventable or treatable.

Yet another widely held fear is that wear and tear of joints inevitably leads to painful arthritis. The cartilage pads that cushion bones do wear down. But less than half the over-65s whose X-rays show the degenerative changes of arthritis suffer symptoms. Many of the aches and pains attributed to acute arthritis may have more to do with weakening muscles than creaky joints. People with some joint damage fare better when they engage in regular and moderate exercise such as walking or swimming.

This is not to say that ageing is a benign process – the immune system starts to decline at around 30, metabolism slows from 25 onwards, eyesight declines in the 40s, bone mass reaches its peak in the 30s and it's downhill from then – particularly post-menopause for women. What is apparent, however, is that ageing need not be the disastrous and burdensome process that it often seems and one that is certainly open to redefinition.

Promoting health and well-being in the elderly is a priority for health promotion. The goals are obvious – healthier life-styles (diet, exercise, non-smoking, sensible drinking, etc.), more involvement in the community, a sense of identity, economic security, all of which are laudable objectives. What can trends tell us about the ways the mechanisms by which these goals can be attained? Using Naisbett's maxim that you need to understand the present to predict the future, what is happening now that might suggest trends that may have an impact on promoting the health of elderly people?

Florida is a State which tends to lead social innovation, it is also a State which has a greater proportion of elderly people. Demographically, it already looks like the USA of 1995. Already in Florida, there are signs of an age war: younger people see their social security payments going to the 'wealthy' elderly, and some communities outlaw residents under 19 to ensure peace and quiet. Whatever the reality or outcome of the age war, there are distinct signs of a grey revolution gathering force in Florida and other states.

Spending Power
Americans over 50 earn more than half the discretionary income in the country. The Information Society megatrend cannot avoid the age market. The trend towards specialist journals and magazines is leading to a burgeoning of glossy special interest publications. Major firms are forming special groups to study the 'senior market'. *Time* (22 February 1988) reported that 'we have designed America to fit the size, shape and style of a country we used to

be, and what we used to be is young'. Books and newspapers, with their tiny print, are designed for young, wide eyes, as is the lighting in public places. Buttons, jars and door knobs are obstacles to those with arthritis. Traffic lights are timed for a youthful pace.

Grey Power

For years politicians have viewed the aged as a uniform group – physically and often mentally feeble, politically compliant, socially inert. Any politician/presidential candidate who makes this assumption is now at risk from grey pressure groups. The American Association of Retired Persons (AARP), with 8 million members is bigger than many countries. The Grey Panthers, with 80,000 members, pressures Congress on everything from health insurance to housing costs. In 1988 the formidable grey lobby has moved full force into grass roots, presidential politics. The AARP in the New Hampshire primary produced a booklet called 'You Can Select A President', a brash promise until you consider that only 101,000 Democrats voted in the primary in 1984 and the AARP has 145,000 members in New Hampshire. In San Francisco, Grey Panthers have campaigned on AIDS, against aid to the Contras in Languna Beach and for Robert Dole in the New Hampshire primary. Grey power is becoming a political force to be reckoned with.

Grey Living

With all the brashness of its youth-oriented culture, America is finding a new way to grow old. Far from fading away, the elderly seem to be brightening on the horizons of the mind, the family, the workplace and the community. No longer are Americans retiring gracefully; corporations and charities are now finding a deeply skilled, reliable labour force among the growing band of used-to-be and not-ready-to-be retired. Between 1980 and 1986 the number of part-time employees in the USA rose by 23 per cent. The Travellers Insurance Company of Hartford is saving more than $1 million a year by hiring back retired workers instead of paying fees to temporary agencies. Millions of retirees have voluntary jobs in schools, hospitals, prisons and art centres. They are filling the gap left by younger women, once full-time volunteers, who have entered the work force.

Many pensioners are staying healthier, taking more interest in self-care and health promotion, becoming involved in sports and recreation, fulfilling ambitions, travel, education, surfing, mountaineering. Not all aged Americans are, or can be, involved. Divisions are rapidly growing between the well and the wealthy, and the poor, sick and often black.

Despite this, the trends are clear for health promotion. Special programmes are needed to reduce inequalities. The major trend in health promotion will be to enrich age, improve quality of life and to provide choice and multiple options (another megatrend) to a group who will be more demanding and in control. For example, uniform retirement age will be a thing of the past and many options, from continued employment to part-time work, consultancy, new careers and paid and unpaid voluntary/care work, will have to come into operation.

The accent in health promotion will be on elderly people taking a greater role in running our society and fulfilling their ambitions. Underlying this will be two factors – growth in preventive education and treatment. A belief that having a role in society and an active body and mind is going to have a much greater impact on health and well-being than the caring services dealing with people who are suffering the inevitable consequences of becoming old. Health promotion will be involved in redefining the meaning of age, retirement, and the political organization of old people.

HIGH-TECH, HIGH-TOUCH

The Healthy City and Megatrends
The WHO (Europe) Healthy Cities Project is a near perfect example of these trends. In many of its tenets it provides an example of an approach that is in line with Naisbett's megatrends. Let us see how well it fits.

Information Society
The development of easy local to global communication means that towns and cities can communicate, and are able to bypass the hierarchy of local: national: international: global. There is an increasing trend for cities to develop cultural and economic relationships that go from the local to the global. Healthy cities represent this trend, whether it is the European Project Group of 24 cities or the many cities around the world that have joined the healthy city movement. The Healthy Cities Project gets cities talking to each other directly, and they are thus able to compare experiences.

Short-term to Long-term
Many aspects of the Healthy Cities Programme demonstrate a movement from the short-term to the long-term, i.e. the ecological approach of the project, and the concentration on the longer-term outcomes of environmental conditions and circumstances on health.

Decentralization
Health in recent times and in many countries has increasingly been seen to be a concern of national government, particularly of government health departments. The Healthy Cities Project breaks down this centralism and returns health to the originators of the old public health, the cities. These are the organizations which are close to the people, and control major aspects of the environment which have an effect on health.

Institutional Help to Self-help
Health for All by the Year 2000[5] and the Healthy Cities Programme recognize the limits of institutional care. It is therapeutic medicine that has had a tendency to centralize in institutions, to improve standards of care and treatment or to gain so-called economies of scale. Traditional public health

never operated on this basis. It was always about public involvement, individuals and community action.

Participation
A key factor in the healthy city approach is the concept of participation. The megatrend is towards a move from representative to participative democracy. Cities are bastions of representative democracy. The healthy city approach will highlight the potential conflict between paternalistic city fathers and people moving into more real participatory activity. The key to the success of the Healthy Cities Project will be the way that it manages to ride the trend of participatory democracy in an organization – the city, rooted in the theory and structures of participation.

Hierarchy to Network
The Healthy Cities Project and movement is in itself a series of networks – national and global networks. The concept of multisectoral working suggests the formation of networks of people in the community and in a variety of relevant organizations, and better communication between departments of the same organization. Multisectoral working requires lateral and diagonal communication of the networks and is also the death nell of the hierarchy.

References

1. Naisbett, J. (1984). *Megatrends: Ten Directions Transforming Our Lives*. Future Macdonald, London.
2. Gibb, N. (1988). Grays on the go. *Time*, February 22, 1988 pp. 42–7.
3. Toufexis, A. (1988). Older but coming on strong. *Time*, February 22, pp. 48–50.
4. Ashton, J., Grey, P. and Barnard, K. (1986). Healthy Cities – WHOs New Public Health Initiative. *Health Promotion* **1** (3), 319–23.
5. World Health Organization (1981). *Global Strategy for Health for All by the Year 2000*. WHO, Geneva.

Creating the New Public Health in One Region

In using a Regional Health Authority and a university department of community health as the base from which to launch the new public health within a region of 2.4 million people, the World Health Organization Strategy of Health For All was taken as the starting point.[1-3] Beginning from a low base of health promotion activity in 1983, an extensive range of initiatives has now been established in the Mersey Region both inside and outside the ambit of the Regional Health Authority. The experience of 5 years of development provides an opportunity to explore the reality of efforts to create a new public health.

The Ecology of the Mersey Region

The Mersey Health Region is geographically the smallest and most compact of the 14 British National Health Service Regions (Fig. 4.1). Administratively the region is coterminous with the counties of Merseyside and Cheshire with six local authorities and ten health districts. With the Mersey estuary and the city of Liverpool at its centre, the region encompasses a cross-section of the nation in the variety of its geographical and physical appearance, in its social structures and activities and in the health of the people it contains and supports; 1 in 20 of the population of England and Wales lives within the Mersey Region, which shows marked contrasts in the conditions of life between industrial, urban and rural areas.

To some extent the City of Liverpool and its surrounding districts dominate the region. From its modest beginnings as a fishing village on the River Mersey, Liverpool's history has reflected and anticipated that of much of the rest of the region and of the country. Liverpool's commercial growth effectively dates from the late seventeenth century, although most of its fabric dates from the nineteenth century and later. In the aftermath of the Victorian age when the city of Liverpool was founded on the slave-trade and the opening

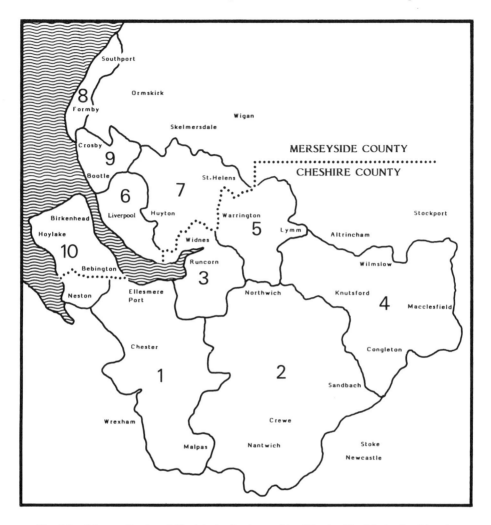

Fig. 4.1. Mersey Regional Health Authority and its District Health Authorities. 1, Chester; 2, Crewe; 3, Halton; 4, Macclesfield; 5, Warrington; 6, Liverpool; 7, St Helens and Knowsley; 8, Southport and Formby; 9, South Sefton; 10, Wirral.

of the sea routes to the Empire, we in the twentieth century are left with the decaying remnants of the obsolete docklands, an infrastructure of inner-city deprivation, appalling unemployment rates and newly created social problems in the form of overspill estates where social relations have been fragmented.[4-7]

In the nineteenth century under the boom-town conditions which prevailed and the immigration of tens of thousands of destitute Irish men and women fleeing from the potato famine and assisted by poverty and malnutrition, epidemic infectious diseases were rampant. At that time, Liverpool was identified as the most unhealthy town in the country in which to live. It was on account of the appalling health statistics and social conditions that the Town Council appointed William Henry Duncan as the first Medical Officer of Health in the country in 1847.[8]

The current recession and major structural changes in the economy have served to further disadvantage an area in no position to cope with many of its existing problems. Riots in the city in 1981 focussed international attention on the city and on the unhealthiness of an environment characterized in part by squalor, poverty, unemployment and inadequate education. In contrast, Cheshire, despite its close connection with the great manufacturing counties of the north and the fact that in the north and east the cotton districts extend across its borders, is on the whole an agricultural county, being particularly renowned for dairy farming and the manufacture of dairy products. The county town of Chester with its quiet prosperity provides a sharp comparison with the Mersey conurbation.

One major structural development in the past 20 years has been the designation of Runcorn-Warrington as a New Town to assimilate the overspill population from Liverpool. The main aim in creating a New Town was to provide homes and jobs for 45,000 people and, unlike most of the earlier New Towns, the designated area included an existing town; this created the additional problem of integrating the old with the new.

Overall, the New Town Development can be seen as a large-scale social experiment, whereby in a short time period an essentially Liverpool population has been transplanted from its own environment to a completely new one; the consequences of this for health are incompletely understood.

Developing the New Public Health in Mersey

ORGANIZATIONAL INITIATIVES

The first step was to establish a multidisciplinary Regional Health Promotion Team within the Health Authority along the lines outlined by the Unit for the Study of Health Policy and by Ashton.[9,10] In particular, six underlying principles have been suggested for catalysts of a new public health movement:[10]

1. Activity on health promotion and disease prevention should be carried out at the most decentralized level that is compatible with effective action.
2. There should be a team approach.
3. Participation by the community should be an overriding principle.
4. Health promotion teams should have security of employment and independence of action.
5. A strategic plan for the promotion of health should be produced at the

regional level which is informed by the priorities and objectives decided at the periphery.

6. Health promotion teams should produce annual reports based on the development of appropriate indicators that can be used to assess progress and revise objectives.

The most important initial function of this team was to obtain access to the range of resources which exist within health authorities, and to open up channels of communication for influencing policy making. This group has undergone several changes, the most recent being to incorporate District Health Authority representation, and exclude non-NHS members or officers. The first of these measures should improve the links between the region and the districts, the second resulted from an Authority decision about the nature of the team, which reflects a difficulty in making intersectoral working a reality from a health authority base.

The work programme of the Regional Health Promotion Team (now described as the Health Promotion Management Steering Group) is implemented by a Health Promotion Section under the direction of the Regional Health Promotion Officer in conjunction with the Regional Specialist in Community Medicine (Health Promotion), an academic with an honorary service contract. The regional Health Promotion Officer post is the first of its kind in the UK and is jointly funded by the Health Education Authority and the Mersey Regional Health Authority.

As a sub-committee of the Regional Health Authority, the Health Promotion Management Steering Group has access to both the planning process and programme budgeting. Through the work of the regional Health Promotion Officer and Specialist in Community Medicine, it has also developed a wide range of links with other statutory and non-statutory organizations. In setting about its task the group has drawn freely on lessons to be learned from the public health pioneers of the nineteenth century.

LESSONS FROM THE PIONEERS

A number of important lessons can be learned from pioneers of the old Public Health, notably William Henry Duncan in Liverpool and John Snow in London.[8,11–14] The first is that most public health problems are quite obvious and that indeed they are often staring us quite literally in the face: poor housing and homelessness, unemployment and dangerous work, poverty and inadequate nutrition, pollution of the air, water and food, the brutalization of children growing up in deprived conditions, lack of recreational facilities, poor quality primary health care. Simple ethnography and statistics are usually adequate to define what is happening – in essence, shoe-leather epidemiology.

By and large, medical and other professionals only display an interest in health promotion and prevention when the work can be segmented into identifiable tasks around which can be built requirements for specific knowledge and skills leading to the possibility of charging fees, acquiring salaries and developing career structures. The involvement of the public is not prominent in most professionals' frames of reference; yet this is a prerequisite for a public health movement, one which seeks to include the public in public health.

When Liverpool Town Council appointed Duncan as Medical Officer of Health in 1847 the appointment was not made out of any particular sense of vision. Rather, housing and environmental conditions were so bad that urgent action was deemed to be necessary. Duncan, as a concerned general practitioner, had been the one physician locally with the necessary insight into the living conditions of his patients and the necessary motivation to bring the situation to public attention. He had carried out a survey of the housing conditions of his patients and discovered that about one-quarter of them were living in unventilated, earth-floored cellar dwellings with as many as 16 people to a room and surrounded by squalor. The results of his survey formed the basis of a popular pamphlet and he gave lectures to lay audiences and evidence to the Chadwick Commission on the sanitary conditions of the labouring classes.[15] Duncan recognized the importance of influencing the opinion-formers and policy makers of the day.

Once appointed as Medical Officer of Health Duncan wrote a constant stream of letters to the Board of Health in London drawing their attention to the social conditions in Liverpool and arguing the urgent case for intervention. He produced an annual report for his health committee, thereby helping to make the link of accountability between the task in hand, the work of the public health department and the general public.

Advocacy was seen as an essential part of the work and there was an in-built protection for Duncan's right to free speech. Although when he was appointed in 1847 his initial contract was at the salary of £300 per annum with the right of private practice, this was soon amended to give him a full-time protected position so that he could be truly independent and without any conflict of interest.

Punch, in one of its early issues published in 1847 (Vol. XII, p.44), had some critical comments to make about the salary to be paid by the Liverpool Corporation for the part-time appointment.

> By the papers Mr. Punch learns that the Town Council of Liverpool intend to appoint an Officer of Health, whose duties will consist in the direction of their sanatory arrangements, and whose services they propose to remunerate by a salary of £300 a year, with the liberty to augment that handsome income, if he can, by private practice. Mr. Punch will engage to find a competent person who will willingly undertake the responsibilities of this office, on the liberal terms proposed by the Town Council of Liverpool.
>
> Mr. Punch, on behalf of the respectable medical gentleman, his nominee, will promise that he, the said respectable medical gentleman, shall devote his full attention to his official duties, and endeavour to

make money by private practice only at those few leisure moments when he shall have nothing else to do. For, although a practitioner of any eminence expects, generally, to make at least a thousand a year, this gentleman shall regard his situation, bringing him in £300, as of primary importance, and shall look upon his private earning as matters of secondary considerations.

If the Officer of Health recommended by Mr. Punch shall have for a patient a rich butcher, with a slaughter house in a populous neigh-bourhood, an opulent fellmonger or tallow-chandler, with a yard or manufactory in heart of town, he shall not hesitate from motives of interest to denounce their respective establishments as nuisances. He shall not fail to point out the insalubrity of any gas-works, similarly situated, the family of whose proprietor he may attend; and if any wealthy old lady who may be in the habit of consulting him shall infringe the Drainage Act, he shall not fail to declare the circumstances to the authorities. (Quoted in Frazer, W.M., 1947, *Duncan of Liverpool*, Hamish Hamilton, London.)

Advocacy was seen as an essential part of the work and medical officers of health in England could only be sacked for professional incompetence; not for making statements which might be politically unpalatable.

This health advocacy function was largely lost in the United Kingdom when, in 1974, preventive medicine became the responsibility of centrally appointed Health Authorities rather than locally elected municipal councils, and the community physicians came increasingly to be seen as medical civil servants who should be uncontroversial. With a few notable exceptions the Community Health Councils which were established to represent the public interest have been unable to fill the void. More outspoken community physicians have found themselves in trouble with their authorities for lobbying in favour of seat-belt legislation or opposing tobacco marketing practices. Recent examples include that of a doctor who was suspended from his work for suggesting that condom machines should be provided in sixth-form colleges and another for criticizing the reduction of family planning services. Clearly, an unfettered health advocacy and free debate is a precondition of public participation and effective public health action. There has been a growing interest in the revival of annual reports and this is one of the positive recommendations to come out of the recent Acheson committee enquiry into public health in England.[16]

Public health needs to be pragmatic and opportunistic, perhaps taking action before causal links have been clarified and in defiance of the prevailing scientific orthodoxy. John Snow, in the nineteenth century, insisted that the handle be removed from the water pump in Broad Street 20 years before the true causes of cholera were established. People who advise the public about health have to offer an informed view which leads to appropriate action based on prudence, and a holistic understanding which takes into account the multifactorial nature of most health problems. For example, the dairy industry

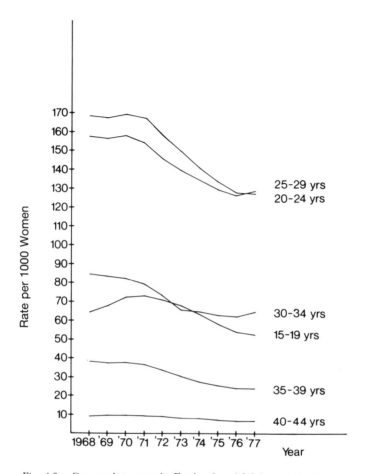

Fig. 4.2. Conception rates in England and Wales, 1968–77.

view that butter has not been shown conclusively to cause heart disease is irrelevant when placed against the fact that increases in consumption of dairy products have been associated with increased heart disease and a great deal of indirect evidence to suggest a causal association.

Riding established trends can help in a sensible use of resources, and also give public health a high and positive profile. When the handle was taken from the Broad Street pump, the cholera epidemic had already passed its peak, but it was public health that received the credit. It isn't cynical to recognize the importance of having an understanding of the natural history of public health phenomena and of working with them in a creative way.

With many behaviour-related health problems there is a one-generation lag between behaviour change and adaptive response by both individuals and society. This can be seen, for example, by reference to pregnancy and induced abortion rates during the past 20 years. A change in social attitudes to sexual behaviour led initially to an increase in unplanned pregnancy and abortion. This prompted the wider availability of contraceptive services (in 1974 in England and Wales) and a falling rate of conception which was most marked in older age groups at first and only later among younger women (Fig. 4.2). Between-country comparisons of the rate of decline in teenage conception gives a good indication of the extent to which policy changes in the form of relationships education and birth control, and youth counselling services have been responsive to the needs of young people and supportive of their desire to behave in a responsible way. Whereas teenage conception rates in Sweden and Denmark fell by 40 per cent in 1970–86, that in England and Wales fell by only 15 per cent and that in the United States actually increased.[17]

Existing trends which would show benefit from a supportive public health response at the present time include action on smoking and nutrition-related diseases, on drink-driving and the provision of high-quality screening services for cancer of the breast, bowel, cervix and testis.

Both Duncan and Snow were not shy of controversy and were willing to stand up and argue with the establishment of the day – they were in effect trouble makers for health or health advocates.

Health Promotion in the Mersey Region

AGENDA SETTING

The Mersey Regional Health Promotion Team has developed a Strategy for Health Promotion which is intended to result in a systematic approach throughout the ten districts which make up the region.[2] This strategy is based on the British Government publication *Care in Action* and on the World Health Organization Strategy of Health For All.[1,18] The strategy takes account of some of the important lessons from the past in trying to create a healthier future.

A central part of preparing the groundwork of the strategy was recognized to be agenda setting for key opinion formers and decision takers within the Mersey Region. It was felt that despite the 10 years of discussion about preventive medicine which had taken place in developed countries since the publication of the Lalonde report in Canada and the series of prevention-orientated reports which had followed it, confusion persisted at a local level as to what Health Authorities and other statutory and voluntary bodies should actually be doing.[19–21]

In addition, there seemed to be considerable ignorance of the wider context including that of the strategy of Health For All. It was felt that if there was to be any real prospect of developing a multisectoral approach to health promotion based on public participation and the extended concept of primary health care described by Vuori, it would be necessary to produce a document which placed local health data firmly in the local context but which drew clearly on the WHO strategy.[22] The audience for the document was to be local politicians, members of Health Authorities, members of Community Health Councils and Local Authorities, the active members of local community groups and charities with a health interest and health staffs of all kinds within the region.[23,24]

COMMUNITY DIAGNOSIS

The reference point for almost all the Mersey health promotion initiatives has been the community diagnosis which was produced in 1983/4, *Health in Mersey – A Review* [23] This 91-page document was a descriptive and analytical assessment of the state of health of people in the Mersey region with comparisons between the ten districts. In essence it was a Local Lalonde and Black Report. The compilation of the report involved collaboration between the Regional Health Authority Statistics Department and The Department of Community Health at the University of Liverpool Medical School. It also required the identification of essential non-health services databases such as those relating to education, social services and the police, and the collection of such data which was not routinely used by the health authority (Table 4.1).

Additional analyses were carried out by the Regional Health Authority Statistics section to refine the data for presentation, to enable district comparisons to be made, and to construct novel indices such as the standard years of life lost ratio (prior to age 75).

Table 4.1   Types and sources of data used in the production of *Health in Mersey – A Review* [23]

Type of data	Source (no. of organizations)
Census data related to living and working conditions	OPCS/RHA/County Councils (2) Local District Authorities (13)
Fertility and mortality statistics	
Hospital morbidity data	(HAA) Regional Health Authority
Family doctor preventive medical services and other family doctor data	Family Practitioner Committees (5)
Health Authority preventive medical services	
Community Health manpower and resources	District Health Authorities (10)
Special educational needs data	Local Education Authorities (5)
Road traffic deaths, narcotic and other offences	Merseyside and Cheshire County Constabularies
Chronic sickness and disability data	Social Services (5) Local Authorities (6)
Consumer interests	Community Health Councils (11)

Table 4.2 Contents of *Health in Mersey – A Review*[23]

Chapter 1 The nature of the health field
Chapter 2 Defining the problem. The determinants of health
Chapter 3 Health in Mersey – The ecology of the region
Chapter 4 The population of Mersey health region
Chapter 5 The causes of death and ill-health
Chapter 6 Prevention or cure – The development of a strategy for health promotion
Chapter 7 Health for all by the year 2000
Chapter 8 Twelve priorities for Mersey.
Chapter 9 A strategy for action, including information and research needs

It is a common experience that once information systems have been established, disproportionate amounts of time are often spent in collecting statistical data compared with the time which is spent examining its meaning; much of the output consists of volumes of tables which accumulate on shelves, untouched by human thought and consequently the data itself is frequently of progressively reducing quality through lack of feedback to collectors and collators. The exercise of producing a report was intended to identify what data was available as well as what was missing and to synthesize information from different databases of relevance to health promotion.

The outcome of the work was a report written in a style which would be easily understood by the informed lay reader, with much of the material being presented visually in the form of diagrams and figures. The report was intended to present a historical and ecological account of health within the region, and to highlight the major causes of premature death and disability and the priorities for health promotion at each stage of the human life-cycle (Table 4.2).

From a review of the state of health within the region and the discussion of health strategies in other countries, 12 priority topics for health promotion in Mersey emerged (Table 4.3). For each of these topic areas a section was

Table 4.3 Priorities for *Health in Mersey – A Review*[23]

1. Planned parenthood
2. Control of sexually transmitted disease
3. Antenatal care including genetic screening
4. Improved child health and increased immunization uptake
5. The prevention of death and disability from accidents and environmental causes
6. Improved dental health
7. Some specific aspects of life-style related to premature death (including diet, exercise, stress, tobacco, alcohol and drugs)
8. The effective control of high blood pressure
9. Early detection of cancer
10. Reduction of disability in the elderly
11. Dignity and comfort at the time of death
12. A healthy mind and healthy body. Positive health, especially as it relates to a health strategy for young people

written which attempted to synthesize the necessary action for a concentrated approach to health promotion. The resources and expertise available for health promotion within the region were reviewed, and the facilitating and hindering factors identified where this was possible.

This document has played a part in two processes: it has informed the strategies developed by the Regional and District Health Authorities but, perhaps more powerfully, has informed the public, both directly and indirectly.

HANDLING THE REPORT

The report was launched at the first Mersey Health Promotion Conference, a one-day event attended by 550 opinion formers and decision takers from around the region. They included Health Authority members and officers, local politicians and officers, interested professionals, non-governmental organizations with an interest in health promotion, and the mass media. The programme included a range of scene-setting presentations from around the country, defining the scope for prevention and health promotion, with examples of good practice. It was intended that participants would return to their organization or district, primed to ask questions about what needed to be done and what was actually happening. In this way the agenda setting for the region would begin.

The conference and the report itself were extensively covered by the mass media. Such has been the interest arising from the report that at the present time 7000 copies have been printed and distributed almost entirely in response to requests. In addition, it has become standard teaching material for medical, health visitor and community nurse students in the region. Subsequently, the report, with its 12 priorities for action, became the basis of a chapter on health promotion in the regional strategic plan, and was incorporated into district planning priorities. More recently, it has become part of both the ministerial and the district review process.

THE REVIEW PROCESS

The review process is intended to provide a non-threatening means of monitoring the implementation of health promotion strategies. Some months in advance of the district reviews, a questionnaire was drawn up based on 12 priority topics for Mersey. In all, some 200 questions were asked, defining what activities were being pursued in each district in relation to these topics. It was felt to be important only to ask questions to which at least some of the districts could respond affirmatively, making the exercise a positive one. Replies from the 10 districts were collated and laid out in a way which made comparison easy. These were made available for discussion within the districts, and provided the basis for the District Review meetings. Agreement has been negotiated between the region and each district on specific initiatives to be taken over the next 12 months.

The intention behind the report was to make a start, and it seems to have had that effect. The strength of the positive response towards the original report from around the region would seem to indicate that even if health workers have sometimes been slow to appreciate the importance of health promotion and prevention, the general public and their representatives are in little doubt about it.

Consciousness Raising – the bottom-up approach

Technical briefing of opinion formers and decision takers is necessary for a health promotion strategy to succeed, but is not of itself sufficient. A parallel process of consciousness-raising on a large scale, leading to more informed individual and collective actions to improve health and the incorporation of health promotion ideas into the political process from the ground up, is equally important.

The underlying expectation is that by mobilizing the public through increased knowledge and changes in attitude and understanding, leading to a greater confidence in public participation in health, individuals can become in a sense their own health experts. The collective effect of such a phenomenon should be a major improvement in public health as a result of individual healthy choices, supported by increasingly responsive and healthy public policies at a local and national level.

The tendency has been to see consciousness-raising as being about campaigns in the mass media but, in recent years, it has become clear that such campaigns in isolation have little chance of achieving long-term effects. There has been a growing realization that Lalonde's concept of influencing the entire health field in which health choices are shaped is necessary for real progress.[19] One element of such an approach is the health fair as an opportunity for active learning.[25]

THE HEALTH PROMOTION FAIR

The International Garden Festival, held in Liverpool from April to October 1984, offered a unique opportunity to bring health-related information to a mass audience as part of Mersey Regional Health Authority's health promotion strategy.

Health was made a major theme throughout the festival and educational material was featured in a number of areas within the site, including the area containing allotment and other horticultural gardens. The term 'health fair' was used to denote the range of activities rather than a single static base, and the objective was to provide active learning. Activities included static displays, providing information on a range of health matters; dynamic displays, consisting of health-orientated activities such as aerobic dancing, yoga, meditation and sports; and public participation, involving physical fitness testing and interactive computerized life-style assessment.

Of the 3.3 million people who attended the International Garden Festival, 250,000 were estimated to have attended the static part of the fair, and most of them made use of the computerized life-style assessment; 11,000 actually took a fitness test. Software was especially developed for computer analysis of life-styles and fitness, and this has subsequently been in steady demand from both home and abroad.

Computerized Life-style Assessment
Twelve computers offered a range of self-operated programs which included a dental health game, an actuarial assessment of longevity and an interactive life-style analysis. The life-style analysis provided a printout for each individual giving advice on their life-style. The areas included in the program were diet, smoking, weight, stress, alcohol intake and heart disease risk.

Fitness Testing
The health promotion assistants received training during a 2-week induction period. This consisted of:

1. Education on major health problems and the relationships to life-style.
2. Instruction in fitness testing and the interpretation of results.
3. Instruction in the use of computer facilities.
4. Advice on communication and presentation to the public.

The venue was constantly manned using a rota system, with additional numbers present on weekends and bank holidays. The fitness tests used were:

1. *Stamina test*: heart rate was measured, using a Cardionics Cardiometer, during the final minute of a 6-minute bout of submaximal exercise on a stationary cycle ergometer.
2. *Grip strength*: a hand grip Dynometer (British Indicators) was used. Three grip attempts were made with each hand and the best score for each hand used.
3. *Flexibility*: measured using a sit and reach bench.
4. *Body fat*: skinfold fat was measured at four body sites – subscapularis, supra-iliac, triceps and umbilical – from which the percentage of body fat was calculated (Harpenden Skinfold Calipers).

The data were entered on a computer (Commodore 64) and scores were generated by comparisons with the norms and percentiles from the Canadian Public Health Project.[26]

Twelve months after the initial interview a sample of 234 people who had completed a research questionnaire at the time of their initial contact were sent a further questionnaire to complete themselves. With a response rate of 67 per cent the major finding was that there appeared to have been actual changes in behaviour in the three main topics of the health fair, i.e. diet, smoking and exercise (24 per cent had an improved diet, 20 per cent were taking more exercise and 6 per cent were smoking less or had stopped).

An important aspect of health promotion which this programme illustrates is the value of initiatives which combine mass coverage with an individual approach. This satisfies the requirements of public health while keeping the satisfaction and quality which goes with an individual service. In this case it was possible by using a combination of unskilled workers and high-technology microcomputers – high-tech and high-touch.

In a sense, part of the hidden health promotion agenda was to provide positive work experience for 56 long-term unemployed people who were recruited to staff the health fair as a part of a Manpower Services Commission Community (job creation) Programme. The staff had the opportunity to be part of a friendly, task-orientated work-group with a great deal of public contact and potential job satisfaction. In addition, they gained a great deal of health knowledge for themselves and, indirectly, for their families. A high proportion of the staff obtained work during the period of the scheme, and some returned to study having found renewed self-confidence and motivation. Arrangements were made for staff to receive details of National Health Service vacancies which occurred while they were on the scheme.

The importance of an emphasis on personal development in such schemes as part of a health promotion strategy was self-evident, and efforts are now being made to extend the possibilities through scheme exchanges with other countries. Job creation is, in itself, a health promotion priority in an area where some local government wards have as many as 80 per cent of the adult males unemployed.

The success of the Garden Festival health fair can be assessed in one way by its expansion to employ 130 people working from five mobile double-decker buses by the time the festival ended.

OTHER ASPECTS OF CONSCIOUSNESS-RAISING

The opportunistic use of publicity and of the mass media presents creative opportunities to reach a large audience at low cost, and Mersey provides a number of examples.

The transformation of the Dr Duncan's pub in Liverpool into a public health theme pub was based on the successful experience of Dr Sidney Chave in persuading a London brewery to rename the pub at the site of the Broad Street Pump in Soho in memory of John Snow (Fig. 4.3). The willing cooperation of a Liverpool brewery was obtained and, at the reopening, a local school drama society performed a short Victorian melodrama on the themes of the old and the new public health to a script which they had written themselves. This drama was subsequently produced as a video tape.

Recognizing the importance of mobilizing the social history of the old public health as a reference point for the new, the Health Education Council agreed to fund an annual Duncan lecture. Based in the Liverpool Medical School as a fully-fledged eponymous lecture, with appropriate ceremony, this lecture is intended to provide a platform for the new public health, in the form of an unfolding series of linked lectures. These will continue to develop new public

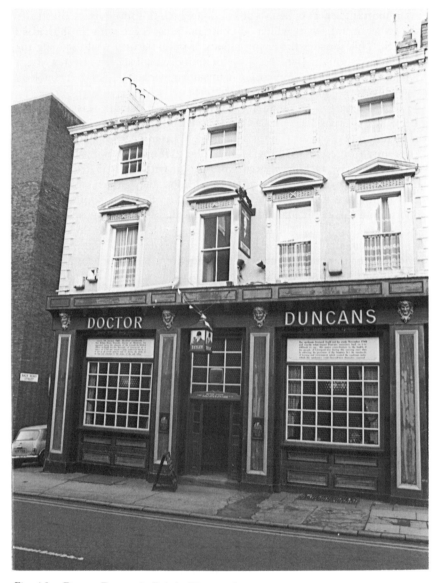

Fig. 4.3.   Doctor Duncan's Pub in Liverpool.

health themes for an audience which on each occasion has consisted of between 200 and 300 people from a wide range of backgrounds, efforts having been made to publicize the lectures well beyond the medical school and university campus.[12,27-30]

Active involvement occurred in the controversy surrounding repeated episodes of water pollution in the area serviced by the North West Water Authority.[31] In this case, it was felt appropriate to host a public meeting in the university in order that an alternative view could be presented to that of the water company.

This is an example of where the university was used as a resource to the local community. It leant legitimacy to public concern and enabled expert opinion to be made directly accessible to the public debate. The issues involved were the inadequacy of arrangements to monitor pollution of the domestic water supply and inform the public, lack of enforcement of the law, lack of accountability of the centrally nominated membership of water authorities and the absence of an independent environmental protection agency.

Health promotion support was publicly withdrawn from the 'Fringe '84' Street Festival as a protest against sponsorship of that event by a tobacco manufacturer, and the Health Promotion Unit made a public protest at the choice of Mersey for test marketing the Skoal Bandit tobacco chewing pouches.

Involvement with Liverpool Football Club was negotiated at no cost, except that of printing posters portraying the squad as a no-smoking team, part of the Health Education Council's Pacesetters Don't Smoke' campaign. Public controversy was generated over the tardiness of milk distributors in the region in responding to consumer demand for doorstep deliveries of fresh skimmed-milk. Collaboration took place with the local commercial radio station to produce a special programme on smoking, which won a gold medal in the international local broadcasting awards. Also, a region-wide competition was run for the 'Slob of the Year' – the most unfit resident who made the greatest progress in becoming fit as a result of involvement with the Health Promotion Unit.

Much of the work was carried out using a mixture of public and private sector funds, mainly through sponsorship where this was felt to be ethically acceptable.

Models of Good Practice

Innovation in large organizations is not an easy matter. According to the diffusion theory of innovation, diffusion takes place as the information about an innovation is disseminated through the appropriate social system and individuals, groups or organizations decide to accept (or reject) the innovation.[32] As more members of the system adopt the innovation an S-shaped diffusion curve is produced, the rate of adoption affecting the steepness of the curve (Fig. 4.4). Stocking has described the limitations to this model when applied to innovations in the British National Health Service including changing patient waking times, preventing rickets in Asians and introduction of the day surgery.[32]

Institutional inertia is the enemy of health promotion. Successful firms have devices to enable them to continue to innovate after their original product champions and charismatic leaders have gone or become complacent.[33] One way to break the cycle of inertia which particularly seems to afflict large

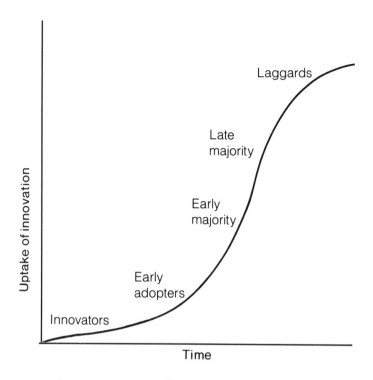

Fig. 4.4. Diffusion of innovations.[32]

bureaucracies is to have local models of good practice.*

Several such models have been developed in Mersey seeking to bring out key principles at the different levels of population and organizational structure (ward, primary health care; district, city and health authorities; region, strategy, policy and research). These models have touched on participation, networking, multisectoral initiatives, use of the mass media, education and training needs, and the political constraints and responses to attempts at innovation among other things. There are a number of examples.

HART – THE HEALTH AND RECREATION TEAM

A Sports Council-funded project, based initially in one health centre, this

---

* 'The main threat to innovation comes from dogs in a manger, they become really dangerous when they get out', i.e. people who are not doing what they should be but are damned if they'll let anybody else do it.

When you try to innovate in a major organization you will be told that you cannot do it. When you ask why not you'll be told that it won't work. When you ask if its been tried they will say no. When you explain that it has been tried elsewhere and that it works you will be told that it won't work here. When you ask why you will be told that it is all to do with the social history. To understand that it will take a lifetime. The way to break into this cycle of inertia is through local demonstration models of good practice which have taken a risk in being set up.

project was inspired by the Peckham Pioneer Health Centre in pre-war London.[34] That centre was a social experiment which sought to influence the environmental and behavioural determinants of health. The Peckham Health Centre failed to achieve the necessary support for its continuation when the National Health Service was established in 1948, partly because it did not accord with contemporary wisdom about the role of medical care which was seen as becoming increasingly therapeutic.

The sort of comprehensive, social, educational and health centre run on cooperative lines which was pioneered in Peckham is unlikely to be constituted today as a new building. However, it is possible to consider related community resources such as community centres, sports centres and various education and training centres as potentially part of a 'networked health centre' – a functional rather than a physical concept. It should be possible to enter any of these public institutions and readily find the services in the others which are most appropriate to particular needs.

The HART project employs a community development worker to develop these networks, particularly as they relate to sport and exercise, and extensive and active links have now been developed between a number of health and community centres and local government and non-governmental organizations in Liverpool as a result of the project.[35,36] HART has given a considerable boost to the local implementation of the national 'Look After Yourself' programme, has produced a comprehensive local survey of exercise participation, and has developed a number of other initiatives including group outings of women from one health centre for swimming classes at the local baths, rambling for inner-city health centre children in the Welsh mountains, and support for collaborative fun-runs with community groups, thus providing support for community involvement and organization.

MERSEYSIDE DRUGS INFORMATION AND TRAINING CENTRE

This centre is the first of its kind with a Regional Health Authority base. The centre offers a free information service for professional staff and the general public. This includes a wide range of literature on the nature and effects of drug misuse as well as carrying an extensive range of up-to-date research reports. Training is also available, not only for professional workers, but also voluntary and parent support groups.

In view of the unfolding importance of the AIDS epidemic and its relationship to drug abuse, the unit has developed a pioneering programme of harm reduction involving the teaching of safe injection techniques, the provision of clean needles and syringes to intravenous drug users and the distribution of free condoms to drug users and prostitutes.

URBAN HORTICULTURE

In the inner-city areas of the Mersey region, issues of employment, environment, housing, poverty and health converge. The city of Liverpool has lost 25 per cent of its population in the past 15 years, and has an overall adult male unemployment rate which is currently about 26 per cent. Deserted factories, abandoned land and slum housing are characteristic of some of the inner-city wards. The Regional Health Promotion Unit has been collaborating with a community-based housing cooperative, housing associations, the government Task Force and various other agencies to develop a community business based on using derelict land for urban horticulture. This project has given rise to other ideas about the potential for creating new jobs in relation to 'healthy products'.

HEALTHY SUPPLIES AND PRODUCTS

The aim of the project dedicated to healthy supplies and products is two-fold. The first is to use the spending power of the NHS (and other public services) not only to buy locally, but to encourage the creation of new jobs in manufacturing and service industries, especially in areas of high unemployment. This process involves creating links between supply systems, local business, and business and job creation.

The second involves stimulating new business. There would seem to be a growing market for healthy products and services (pure food, healthy and safe furniture, personal and occupational positive health services). One specific aspect of this programme involves the creation of new organizations to market healthy products to the public and 'new' entrepreneurs.

THE MIND, BODY, CITY 'MUSEUM'

A development of the health fair, the Mind, Body, City Museum or Body, Mind, Magic is a joint project under discussion between the Mersey Regional Health Authority and Merseyside Development Corporation intended to draw in the leisure industry and commercial organizations. The museum would be a cross between a science centre and a theme park. It would aim to give people a powerful and enjoyable insight into the working of their own bodies and minds, and the environment best suited to people's talents and potentials. It would use the best ideas and technology of the modern museum and the theme park industry. It would create jobs in an area of high unemployment both in terms of education and its role in improving the local health environment, economy, and so on. A similar development, 'healthy workplace', is also envisaged, involving a consortium of workplaces. In this project, small business, where most people work and occupational health services are least developed, would be the major focus.

A HEALTH INFORMATION SERVICE

The Mersey Regional Health Promotion Unit has developed a health promotion information service. This information service supports individuals within the region working to set up or develop new health promotion initiatives. Enquirers are helped with up-to-date information and contacts in their areas of interest. The service is seen as complementary to the review process. Negotiations have begun with other regions and interested organizations to see if existing or planned health promotion information services could form a collaborative network, whereby each service would be able to provide the broadest and more cost-effective service to its own clients.

The Limitations of the Health Authority Base

Innovation is never easy, and particular conditions are necessary if it is to be successful. In developing participative, intersectoral health promotion which has a distinctively social entrepreneurial style, there have been many times when a Health Authority has not seemed to be the most appropriate base.

The history of British health authorities lies with hospital management by appointed members, rather than with politically-responsive, broadly-based local initiatives from the Town Hall where the value of intersectoral working could be made more readily apparent. Such was the situation in the United Kingdom prior to 1974, and in Commonwealth countries which have retained the British model of a Local Authority Public Health Department, such as Canada, the potential for developing an effective new public health seems exceptionally rich. Local government in Toronto, for instance, has a political mandate to make Toronto the healthiest city in North America by the year 2000.[37] However, despite the difficulties, there is within the Mersey Region a real commitment to developing health promotion. In this context, new Town Hall-based health promotion initiatives should be seen as complementary rather than competitive.

Lessons from Health in Mersey

According to the Health For All Strategy, the target for information systems is that 'before 1990, member states should have information systems capable of supporting their national strategies for Health For All'. Such information systems should provide support for the planning, monitoring and evaluation of health development and services, assessment of national, regional and global progress towards health for all and dissemination of relevant scientific information; steps should be taken to make health information easily accessible to the public.[38]

The production of the *Health in Mersey Report* was an example of an attempt both to set an agenda for health promotion in the region and to make health information easily accessible to the public. However, during the course of producing the report many of the deficiencies in the present information system became apparent. In particular, it was clear that much routinely collected data of relevance to health promotion was currently not being made use of because it was collected by non-health agencies. In addition, the lack of useful local as opposed to regional or national data, especially in relation to life-styles and preventable risks, highlighted the necessity for new approaches.

As a direct result of this a working party was convened to examine information needs for health promotion within the Mersey Region under the chairmanship of the Chief Statistician of the Regional Health Authority. The terms of reference of the working group were to examine the 12 priority topics for health promotion from the point of view of the information needs in developing the Regional Health Promotion Strategy around them. The approach adopted was essentially that used by the British Health Services Information Steering Group.[39] This consisted mainly of identifying the minimum data sets required to provide information under the following headings:

1. Demand (as a proxy for need).
2. Inputs (resources used or available).
3. Output (workload, population coverage, process and organizational aspects).
4. Outcome (state of health).
5. Environmental (including social, economic and psychological) influences.

The Structure of Information Needs

Five categories of data for Health Promotion could be identified:[40,41]

1. *Health Service data.* Data which is readily available and merely needs to be organized and presented in a useful way.
2. *Related organization data.* Data covering a wide range of organizations from Local Authority to voluntary bodies which is often readily available once arrangements have been made for it to be supplied.
3. *Special survey data.* This forms a significant part of the data needed for health promotion and is likely to be the most costly. Typically, it is needed to describe the local environments which shape healthy choices. The need for such data became repeatedly apparent during the production of the *Health in Mersey* Report. It is needed to supplement currently available routine statistics and enable monitoring of the achievement of health goals to take place. Survey techniques of a 'dipstick' or market research type, allowing periodic assessment of small area based populations, are likely to be the most productive and the piloting of such a technique has already been carried out in relation to shopping habits and coronary prevention in Liverpool.[42]
4. *Analytically derived data.* Typically, this relates to small area statistics for

economic and social variables. Fundamental data are often available (census-based or from national surveys) but it often needs to be analysed in relation to a specific topic or at a specific level of disaggregation.

5. *'Soft' descriptive data.* A complete understanding of each priority topic at a community level requires qualitative data deploying the rich perspectives of anthropology, social and behavioural science.

In reporting the deliberations of the working party a small number of specific indicators have been identified in relation to the 12 priority topics and for each of these its current availability is stated (AN = available now; AR = analysis required; DWR = development work or special survey required). For each of the context statements some survey work will usually be necessary.

The criteria which have been applied for individual indicators are those which have been deployed in the WHO Healthy Cities Project and are as follows:

1. That they should stimulate change by the nature of their political visibility and punch, through being sensitive to change in the short-term and being comparable between cities.*
2. That they should be simple to collect, use and understand, be either directly available now or available in a reasonable time at an acceptable cost.
3. That they should be related to health promotion.[43]

The selection of indicators and targets is not intended to be a final list but a starting point to facilitate the early compilation of comparisons both between and within the Mersey Health Districts. As much as anything they are intended to stimulate debate. The emphasis of the proposed data is on small area comparisons and reduction in equalities. The danger of taking this step is that it may pre-empt the important development and use of health promotion indicators of a type which is not currently available. There is a great need for such new indicators which are centred on the perception, feelings and aspirations of individuals and groups living within our districts. Such complacency is to be resisted. The relationship of the 12 Mersey priorities to the 38 WHO targets is indicated in each case (see Appendix 1).

Part of the development work which is needed for each priority is to enable an accurate description of the context or health field in which the topic itself is but an epiphenomenon; that context must take account of relevant legislation, explicit or implicit public policy and such social, cultural and organizational factors as impinge on people's ability to influence their health status. The

---

* The problem of making health promotion visible as compared with treatment, is well known. It is perhaps best summarized by the story of the two people on a train in Africa. One is standing by the window and periodically throwing a handful of powder out through it. 'What are you doing?' asks the other, 'I'm throwing powder to keep the elephants away', explains the first. 'But there are no elephants', exclaims his companion. 'There you are it works', proclaims the other.

context statement for each priority is best seen as the reciprocal of the health impact statements which need to be made by governmental or non-governmental organizations. With health impact statements the health impact of policies in non-medical sectors is made explicit. Between them, context and health impact statements should provide the bridge of intelligence, monitoring and research for intersectoral action.

It seems likely that one of the consequences of the New Public Health movement will be an increasing recognition of the necessity to develop compatible databases between Local and Health Authorities and other governmental and non-governmental organizations down to the most local levels of population. This needs to be borne constantly in mind.

Health Promotion priorities and suggested indicators and targets for the Mersey Region

PRIORITY 1: PLANNED PARENTHOOD (WHO TARGETS 1–4, 7, 8, 13–17, 18)

Proposed indicators (available now):

- 15–19 year old conception rates,
- proportion of conceptions resulting in a live- or still-birth for age groups 15–19, 20–24, 25–34, 35–44.

Context statement: Availability and characteristics of relationships education (including birth control), accessibility and acceptability of family planning services to all social groups.

Proposed target (No. 1): That by the year 2000 the conception rate for 15–19 year olds in all Districts should be 14/1000 or lower.

Rationale: This level of teenage pregnancy has been achieved in the Netherlands with a broadly similar pattern of teenage sexual activity. As an indicator this statistic is a good summary of the outcome of relationships education and the accessibility and acceptability of family planning services to all social groups.

PRIORITY 2: PREVENTION OF SEXUALLY TRANSMITTED DISEASES (WHO TARGETS 1, 2, 4–6, 10, 13–17, 18)

Proposed indicators (available now):

- gonorrhoea infection rates by sex for age groups 15–19, 20–24, 25–34, 35–44.

Context statement: Availability and characteristics of relationships education (including information about sexually transmitted disease), accessibility and acceptability of genito-urinary treatment services to all social groups.

Note: The numbering of the 12 Mersey Priorities approximates to their place in the life-cycle and not to a league table of priorities.

Proposed target (No.2): That by the year 2000 the increasing trend in gonorrhoea infection rates should have been reversed.

Rationale: Gonorrhoea infection rates can be seen as a tracer of all sexually transmitted disease infection. For the immediate future the numbers of AIDS cases in the region is likely to be insufficient to be used meaningfully at a district or local level. It is probable that as the AIDS epidemic unfolds it will have a similar distribution in place and person as does currently gonorrhoea. The effectiveness of the current initiatives in community-based programmes of health promotion and improvements in the accessibility of treatment services should in the first instance be reflected in stabilized and then declining rates for gonorrhoea infection.

PRIORITY 3: ANTENATAL CARE (WHO TARGETS 1, 2, 4–8, 13–17, 18)

Indicator (available now):

● perinatal mortality rates.

Indicator available with small amount of analysis:

● proportion of infants of low birth weight at a small area level.

Context statement: Availability, accessibility and acceptability of antenatal services including childbirth preparation classes for all social groups.

Proposed Mersey target: That by the year 2000 the proportion of infants of low birth weight in the most disadvantaged ward of the district should be the same as that in the most advantaged ward and the perinatal mortality rates should be similarly equalized.

Rationale: Small area differences in low birthweight and in perinatal mortality rates are predominantly the outcome of social disadvantages manifested directly and indirectly through the effects of poverty on education, nutrition and accessibility to good quality primary health care services. Equalization of the differences in these indicators requires a broad-based attack on the causes through action both in the medical sector and in other sectors which are determined by both local and national public policy. The progressively small numbers involved in perinatal death and the difficulty of demonstrating significant statistical differences between small areas points to the importance of systems of confidential inquiry into any perinatal death. The availability of data on the coverage of antenatal care by 12 weeks from the last menstrual period will provide a tracer on the quality of primary care services to women.

PRIORITY 4: CHILD HEALTH AND IMMUNIZATION (WHO TARGETS 1–5, 7, 13–17, 18)

Indicator (available now):

● immunization coverage levels.

Context statement: Availability, accessibility and acceptability of child health services to all social groups. Extent to which national nutritional standards are met for children in families on low income.

Proposed Mersey target: That by the year 2000 there should be no indigenous measles, poliomyelitis, or congenital rubella.

Rationale: The ability to deliver effectively immunization services to all social groups within the community is a tracer of the quality of all child health services. A secondary target of equalizing social class differences in the height and weight of school leavers should be developed on the basis of the analysis of routinely collected school health service data. The attainment of equalization will depend on broad-based intersectoral policies addressing the issues of national and local nutrition policies, poverty and deprivation.

PRIORITY 5: PREVENTION OF DEATH AND DISABILITY FROM ACCIDENTS AND ENVIRONMENTAL CAUSES (WHO TARGETS 1, 2, 4, 6, 11, 13–17, 18–25)

Indicators (available now):

- number of days NO_x or SO_2 exceed WHO guidelines,
- home ownership by tenure and type,
- proportion of households suffering from overcrowding.

In addition, a variety of indicators on accidents in the home, on the road, at work or sustained during recreation should be available, and a small amount of additional analysis and data on water pollution should be made available with the cooperation of the Water Authorities. Other than this there is a range of development work needed, especially in relation to qualitative indicators of the environment.

Context statements: The existence of fully staffed departments of environmental health in local authorities with adequate mechanisms for public consultation and for liason with health and other relevant agencies.

Proposed Mersey Targets:

1. That by the year 2000 deaths from accidents of all kinds should have been reduced by at least 25 per cent through an intensified effort to reduce traffic, home, occupational and recreational accidents.
2. That by the year 1990 all districts should have fully staffed departments of environmental health in local authorities in accordance with nationally-derived staffing norms. These departments should have adequate mechanisms for public consultation and liaison with health and other relevant agencies.
3. That by the year 1990 a clear picture of chemical pollution risks to the domestic water supply should have been established and a plan drawn up to eliminate it; that measures will have been developed to assess consumer satisfaction with the taste of drinking water and regular consumer surveys begun to be carried out. That by the year 1995 chemical pollution of the

water supply should have ceased to occur and public satisfaction with the taste of drinking water should exceed 95 per cent of the adult population.

4. That by the year 1995 there should be no days in the year on which NO_x or SO_2 levels exceed WHO guidelines.
5. That by the year 1990 the increasing trend of episodes of food poisoning should have been reversed and a system of training courses in the nutritional aspects of food established for food handlers in retail outlets and cafes in both the public and private sector.
6. That by the year 1995 the major known health risks associated with the disposal of hazardous wastes should have been eliminated and bathing beaches within the region should all reach EEC standards.
7. That by the year 2000 the proportion of households suffering from overcrowding in the most disadvantaged ward should be the same as that in the most advantaged ward.
8. That by the year 1995 all employers will have made adequate arrangements to monitor work-related health risks and have agreed a prevention strategy with their work force and with the surrounding population.

Rationale: The environmental area is a central one in health promotion. There is a great need to move from traditional structural indicators which tend to be readily available towards process indicators of environmental quality which need to be developed, particularly through market research techniques. In the bridging period it is appropriate to make as much use of existing data as possible to support the activities of environmental health departments and, in particular, their forming effective intersectoral partnerships and developing meaningful public participation. An example of the effective use of traditional data comes from data linkage of the police and hospital services in Gothenburg to the city engineering and planning departments, where the resulting changes in traffic management and road design have been apparently associated with a significant reduction in road accidents.

PRIORITY 6: DENTAL HEALTH (WHO TARGETS 1–4, 13–18)

Indicator available now with some additional analysis:

- decayed, missing or filled teeth (DMF) profile for 5- and 16-year-olds by sex.

Context statement: Availability, accessibility and acceptability of preventive dental health services to all social groups.

Proposed Mersey Target: That by the year 2000 the DMF ratio at age 5 years in the most deprived ward of the district should be as good as that in the most advantaged.

Rationale: Much improved DMF ratios have been achieved especially in the Scandinavian countries through a public health approach to nutrition policy and to preventive dentistry. The ability to deliver a comprehensive programme for good dental health depends on an acceptance of water fluoridation on the one hand and reduced sugar intake on the other. The attainment of equalization will depend on broad-based intersectoral initiatives addressing all these issues.

PRIORITY 7: SOME SPECIFIC ASPECTS OF LIFE-STYLE RELATED TO PREMATURE DEATH (WHO TARGETS 1–4, 6, 9–19)

Indicators (available now):

- unemployment rates,
- proportion of children receiving free school meals,
- proportion of school leavers continuing into higher education of various types,
- household car ownership,
- premature years of life lost and hospital bed days used by cause.

Context statement: Control over resources related to life-style through time, e.g. accessibility to low-cost, high-quality food for people on low incomes and the possession of the knowledge to take advantage of it.

Proposed Mersey Targets:

1. By the year 2000 mortality from diseases of the circulatory system in people under 65 years of age should be reduced by at least 15 per cent and the death rates in the most disadvantaged ward should be the same as those in the most advantaged.
2. By the year 2000 the current rise in male suicide and attempted suicide rates should be reversed and the decline in female rates should be sustained.
3. By 1990, all districts should have systematic programmes of health education to enhance the knowledge, motivation and skills of people to acquire and maintain health and each school should have at least one teacher designated as having responsibility to co-ordinate health education.
4. By 1995 in all districts there should be established trends in positive health behaviour such as balanced nutrition, non-smoking, appropriate physical activity and good stress management. Indicators of these trends should be available at ward level and the differences between the most advantaged and disadvantaged wards in health knowledge and behaviour and biological status should be narrowing.
5. By 1995 in all districts there should be established downward trends in health-damaging behaviour such as overuse of alcohol and pharmaceuticals, use of illicit drugs and dangerous chemical substances, dangerous driving and violent social behaviour. Indicators of these trends should be available at ward level and the differences between the most

advantaged and disadvantaged wards in health knowledge and behaviour and biological status should be narrowing. By the year 2000 the proportion of the population living in the most disadvantaged ward and engaged in satisfying work should be the same as that of people living in the most advantaged ward.

Rationale: The life-styles area is a central one in health promotion. There is a great need to move away from traditional indicators of mortality and morbidity, which tend to be readily available, towards process indicators of the quality of life which need to be developed especially through market research techniques. In the bridging period it is appropriate to make as much use as possible of existing data to support the work of all those engaged in health promotion to support public participation and the establishment of effective intersectoral partnership.

PRIORITY 8: THE EFFECTIVE CONTROL OF HIGH BLOOD PRESSURE (WHO TARGETS 1–4, 6, 9, 13–17, 18)

Indicator (available now):

● mortality and admission rates from stroke by age and sex.

Context statement: Extent to which stroke prevention is a priority of all agencies, including employers, who are in a relationship with people over age 35. Extent to which protocols of good practice for the detection of hypertension are in effective operation in primary medical care.

Proposed Mersey target: That by the year 2000 death rates from stroke within each district will be reduced by at least 15 per cent among those aged under 75 years, and the death rates from stroke within the most disadvantaged ward will be the same as those in the most advantaged.

Rationale: Mortality and admission rates from stroke as a manifestation of the control of high blood pressure are a tracer of the quality of primary health care services and of their availability to all social groups. Such services include appropriate management tools of primary medical care, such as case-finding, screening and hypertension registers.

PRIORITY 9: EARLY DETECTION OF CANCER (WHO TARGETS 1, 2, 4, 6, 10)

Indicators (available now):

● mortality rates for carcinoma of cervix and breast cancer,
● mortality rates for carcinoma of testis in men,
● mortality rates for carcinoma of bowel and for melanoma in both men and women.

Context statement: Extent to which cancer detection is a priority for all employers and primary medical care teams. Extent to which appropriate systems of information and recall are in place which link the necessary agencies involved in the early detection and treatment of cancer.

Proposed Mersey target: By the year 2000 mortality rates in each district from cancer of the cervix, breast, testis, bowel and skin should be reduced by at least 15 per cent and the mortality rates from each of these cancers in the most disadvantaged ward should be the same as those in the most advantaged ward.

Rationale: Mortality from cancer of the cervix, breast and testis, bowel and skin can frequently be prevented if detected early enough but, at the moment, with the possible exceptions of cancer of the cervix and skin, there is little that can be done in the way of primary prevention. Restrictions of the number of sexual partners and increased condom use during the next few years may have an impact on the incidence of carcinoma of the cervix, and a greater awareness of the dangers of excessive exposure to ultra-violet light may reduce the incidence of skin cancer. Reduction in the case fatality rates from these conditions and equalization of the rates among different social groups depends upon the effectiveness of health education and primary care services in reaching all social groups and in the provision of accessible, acceptable services. The availability of data on the staging of malignancies of each type at the time of diagnosis will further add to our knowledge of the quality of services available in each local area.

PRIORITY 10: REDUCTION OF DISABILITY IN THE ELDERLY (WHO TARGETS 1–4, 6, 9, 11, 12, 13–18)

Indicator (available now):

● permanent sickness levels.

Context statement: Availability of networks of family, friends and caring agencies to provide support and care on the patient's own terms in the place where they would prefer it. Development work needs to be carried out to measure variations in the morbidity load of populations prior to death in relation to the health-promoting characteristics of life-style and environment.

Proposed Mersey target: By the year 2000 permanent sickness levels in the most disadvantaged ward of the district should be as low as those in the most advantaged.

Rationale: Permanent sickness interferes with a person's ability to live a socially, economically and mentally creative life in later years. Measurement of permanent sickness levels in populations is, therefore, an indirect measure of well-being in the elderly. It needs to be complemented by more positive measures of well-being and everyday living assessment which reflect the product of biological ageing and the availability to all social groups of good-quality primary care services aimed at maintaining optimal function.

PRIORITY 11: DIGNITY AND COMFORT AT THE TIME OF DEATH (WHO TARGETS 1, 13, 14, 18)

Indicator (available now):

● none.

Context statement: The climate in which death occurs, whether at home or in an institution. Whether there is a commitment to an open, supportive approach to the management of death which recognizes the needs of patients, relatives, friends and staff and which provides staff with adequate training and support to enable them to fulfil their responsibilities to patients, relatives and friends.

Proposed Mersey target: That by the year 2000 all those dying who are in contact with health and social services should be able to choose where they spend their last days and wherever that is they should be able to expect optimal pain relief, physical comfort and psychological support from professionals.

Rationale: Everybody must die someday. There is a danger of health workers regarding death as a failure rather than seeing its positive management as a challenge. Appropriate measures are needed to ensure that for all social groups dignity and comfort at the time of death is a reality and that the dying, their relatives and friends and their attending health care workers are properly supported.

PRIORITY 12: A HEALTHY MIND IN A HEALTHY BODY – POSITIVE HEALTH (ALL WHO TARGETS, BUT ESPECIALLY 13–17, 18–25)

Indicator (available now):

● none.

This final category of health promotion in the Mersey Region is a healthy mind in a health body, i.e. positive health. This category is intended to complement the more traditional perspective of most of the other 11 categories with their biomedical or biosocial emphasis. It is intended to underline the essential wholeness of health as 'a resource for everyday life'.

A healthy life is more than life without disease and disability. Health is a positive asset which gives people, families, groups and society the ability to lead productive and satisfying lives both as individuals and as members of a community. Health promotion is seen as the process of enabling people to increase control over and to improve their health; it involves the population as a whole in the context of everyday life rather than focussing on people at risk for specific diseases.

Important aspects of this approach include a focus on the determinants of health and on the use of diverse but complementary methods based on meaningful public participation. For health promotion to be effective it is important to develop healthy public policies and for professionals to take on the important role of enabler in their work with individuals and groups. Through these means it is possible to strengthen communities based on the widespread acquisition of personal knowledge and skills in the context of environments which support choice.[45]

Statistics which measure positive health in a meaningful way are not readily available. Traditional census indicators of housing, physical environment and social and occupational status give some clues. Such measures need to be supplemented by those which can give people-centred assessments of psychological, social and physical well-being at a small area level and which tackle the difficult questions of the extent to which people feel that they have power over their own lives and can participate fully in community life.

The development of community survey methods for measures of this kind is a priority in monitoring the health of the population. Such methods may grow out of the use of existing instruments, such as the Nottingham Health Profile, or may depend on new approaches and developments, e.g. the repertory grid technique based on personal construct theory.

The context in which these kinds of measures will be developed is one in which there is widespread acceptance of the need to go beyond narrow physical and biological measures of health and to embrace psychological and social measures in order to obtain a complete picture. In turn, such a paradigm shift implies a recognition of the sovereignty of people's own perceptions of their health and of the necessity to develop a new partnership between the public and professionals engaged in health work. (Availability status – DWR.)

WHO targets 26–31 (appropriate care with the emphasis on primary health care) and targets 32–37 (research planning, information and education) apply to all 12 Mersey priorities.

Proposed Mersey target: That by the year 2000 the ability of people living in the most disadvantaged ward of the district to lead a socially and economically productive life should be the same as those living in the most advantaged ward.

Rationale: Target 12 subsumes all the WHO targets and the 11 Mersey priorities. It is but the essence of positive healthy as a resource for everyday life. At the moment there are no entirely suitable indicators available, although some survey instruments are available which provide clues. The development of market research approaches to people-centred survey work is a priority in clarifying the extent to which social health is being achieved for all social groups.

Underpinning all 38 WHO targets and all 12 Mersey Region Health Promotion priorities are the necessity to reorientate medical care towards health promotion and primary health care; to develop appropriate education, training and research support for health promotion through collaboration of whichever educational and research establishments are most appropriate; to make appropriate management and planning arrangements, based on appropriate health information systems, to ensure the effective and efficient deployment of scarce resources, and to develop local, national and international policies which support health promotion based on public participation and intersectoral collaboration at the local level.

The identification of necessary policy initiatives and their representation to governmental and non-governmental organizations through health advocacy is a responsibility of all those engaged in health promotion work.

The targets outlined above are based on their relevance to the 12 health promotion priorities for the Mersey Region and the readiness of availability of supportive indicator data in the immediate future or medium term. In addition, the stimulant effect on health promotion processes is an important spin-off from the early visibility of the effects of action as reflected in some of the suggested data.

Implications of the Work in Mersey

The Health For All Strategy and the Mersey Region Health Promotion strategy provide the starting point for a consideration of the information needs of effective health promotion work. It is apparent that there already exists a range of indicators which can be used to help establish meaningful and motivating targets to be reached between now and the year 2000. It is also apparent that the currently available data, both quantitative and qualitative, have limitations and that development work needs to be carried out as a matter of urgency.

Mechanisms need to be established so that databases for a variety of sectors and agencies are automatically linked and made use of; new information giving social information about public perceptions and aspirations as well as describing those processes which mediate in health promotion needs to be collected, drawing on market research and other techniques developed in social and behavioural science and in the business world. Economic assessment of the costs and benefits of either achieving or not achieving the targets needs to be carried out. Biennial health for all reports structured around the Mersey targets and indicators will need to be compiled.

One useful approach to the implementation of policies designed to achieve a specific target is to establish a working group with a specific brief to report back with recommendations for action based on the health for all philosophy. An example of such an approach has been the development of an exercise policy in the Mersey Region.

References

1. World Health Organization (1981). *Global Strategy for Health For All by the Year 2000*. WHO, Geneva.
2. Ashton, J. and Seymour, H. (1985). An approach to health promotion in one region. *Community Medicine*, **7**, 78–86.

3. Ashton, J., Seymour, H., Ingledew, D., Ireland, R., Hopley, E., Parry, M., Ryan, M. and Holbourn, A. (1986). Promoting the new public health in Mersey. *Health Education Journal.* **45** (3), 174–9.
4. Lane, T. (1986). *Liverpool – Gateway of Empire.* Lawrence and Wishart, London.
5. Hayes, M.G. (1987). *Past Trends and Future Prospects.* City of Liverpool Planning Department, Liverpool.
6. Evans, E.S.P. (1977). *City in Transition.* City of Liverpool Planning Department, Liverpool.
7. Redfern, P. (1982). *Profile of our Cities in Population Trends,* No. 30. HMSO for OPCS, London.
8. Frazer, W.M. (1947). *Duncan of Liverpool.* Hamish Hamilton, London.
9. Dennis, J., Draper, P., Griffiths, J., Partridge, J., Popay, J., Alderslade, R., Bartley, D., Chambert, J., Hunter, D., Knight, H., Mair, H. and Zealley, H. (1979). *Rethinking Community Medicine.* A report from a study group. USHP, Guys Hospital Medical School, London.
10. Ashton, J.R. (1982). Towards prevention – an outline plan for the development of health promotion teams. *Community Medicine* **4**, 231–7.
11. Duncan, W.H. (1843). *The Physical Causes of the High Rate of Mortality in 1843.* Quoted in W.M. Frazer, *op.cit.*
12. Chave, S.P.W. (1984). Duncan of Liverpool – and some lessons for today. *Community Medicine* **6**, 61–71.
13. Snow, J. (1985). *On the Mode of Communication of Cholera,* 2nd edition. Churchill, London.
14. Chave, S.P.W. (1955). John Snow – The Broad Street pump and after. *The Medical Officer* **99**, 347–9.
15. Chadwick, E. (1842). *The Sanitary Condition of the Labouring Population of Great Britain.* Republished (1965, ed. M.W. Flinn) by Edinburgh University Press, Edinburgh.
16. Acheson, E.D. (1988). *Public Health in England.* HMSO, London.
17. Jones, E.F., Forrest, J.D., Goldman, N., Henshaw, S., Lincoln, R., Rosoff, J.I. and Westoff, D. (1986). *Teenage Pregnancy in Industrialized Countries (The Guttmacher Report).* Yale University Press, New Haven and London.
18. HMSO (1981). *Care in Action.* HMSO, London.
19. Lalonde, M. (1984). *A New Perspective on the Health of Canadians.* Ministry of Supply and Services, Canada.
20. HMSO (1979). *Prevention and Health: Everybody's Business.* HMSO, London.
21. Robbins, C. (ed.) (1984). *Health Promotion in North America; Lessons for the United Kingdom.* Kings Fund, London.
22. Vuori, H. (1984). Primary health care in Europe – problems and solutions. *Community Medicine* **6**, 221–31.
23. Ashton, J. (1984). *Health in Mersey – A Review.* Liverpool Univeristy Department of Community Health, Liverpool.
24. Ashton, J. (1984). Health in Mersey – an exercise in community diagnosis. *Health Education Journal* **44**, 178–80.
25. Hussey, R.M., Edwards, M.B., Reid, J.A., Sykes, K., Seymour, H., Hopley, E. and Ashton, J.R. (1987). Evaluation of the International Garden Festival Health Fair. *Public Health* **101**, 111–17.
26. Canadian Public Health Project (1979). *Standardized Test of Fitness Norms and Percentile Scores.* The Minister of State, Canada.
27. Godber, G.E. (1986). Medical Officers of Health and Health Services. *Community Medicine* **8** (1), 1–14.

28. Hellberg, H. (1987). Health For All and Primary Health Care in Europe. The Third Duncan Lecture. *Public Health* **101,** 151–7.
29. Acheson, E.D. (1988). On the State of the Public Health. The Fourth Duncan Lecture. *Public Health* **102,** 431–37.
30. Player, D. (1988). The Politics of Public Health. The Fifth Duncan Lecture. *Public Health* **103** (4), 263–79.
31. Ashton, J. (1985). Pollution of the water supply in Mersey and Clwyd – a cause for concern. *Community Medicine* **71,** 299–303.
32. Stocking, B. (1985). *Initiative and Inertia. Case Studies in the NHS.* Nuffield Provincial Hospitals Trust, London.
33. Peters, T.J. and Waterman, R.H. (1982). *In Pursuit of Excellence – Lessons from America's Best-run Companies.* Harper and Row, New York.
34. Ashton, J. (1977). The Peckham Pioneer Health Centre: a reappraisal. *Community Health* **8,** 132–7.
35. Ireland, R. (1985). Health and Recreation Team (HART): Mersey Regional Health Authority Phase One Monitoring Report – Establishing the Project. Sports Council Research Unit, Manchester.
36. The Sports Council (1988). Participation Demonstration Projects – Health and Recreation Team (HART): Mersey Regional Health Authority Phase 2 Monitoring Report. Sports Council Research Unit, Manchester.
37. Ashton, J., Grey, P. and Barnard, K. (1986). Healthy Cities – WHO's New Public Health initiative. *Health Promotion* **1** (3), 319–24.
38. World Health Organization (1985). *Targets in Support of the European Strategy for Health For All.* WHO, Copenhagen.
39. Korner, E. (1982). *Steering Group on Health Services Information. First Report to the Secretary of State.* HMSO, London.
40. Ashton, J. (ed.) (1987). *Indicators and Targets for 'Health For All' in the Mersey Region.* Department of Community Health, Liverpool University Medical School, Liverpool.
41. Ashton, J. (1988). *Tying Down the Indicators and Targets for Health For All* (in press).
42. Brackpool, J., Ramharry, S. and Ashton, J. (1985). *Shopping and Coronary Prevention in Liverpool – A Pilot Study.* Liverpool University Department of Community Health, Liverpool.
43. World Health Organization (1987). *The Healthy Cities Project: A Proposed Framework for City Reports* (eds Barnard, K. and Itani, H.). Discussion Paper for the WHO Healthy Cities Symposium. Dusseldorf, June 1987. WHO, Copenhagen.
44. World Health Organization (1984). *Health Promotion: A Discussion Document on the Concepts and Principles.* WHO, Copenhagen.
45. World Health Organization, Health and Welfare, Canada and Canadian Public Health Association (1986). *The Ottawa Charter for Health Promotion.* WHO, Copenhagen.

5 Populism

Dilemmas

There are a number of dilemmas which invariably face the practitioner of health promotion, dilemmas which have been generated from the historical, professional and organizational roots of the activity. These dilemmas include:

1. *Health is not primarily under the control or direct influence of the health service.* Health and all its accoutrements (knowledge, affect, skills, example and environment) are on the whole not gained or lost in hospital or through health care. Health care organizations do not usually build houses, construct road systems, own art galleries, operate supermarkets or recreation and leisure services. Health is gained, lost and maintained in the real worlds of work, home, leisure and daily life.

2. *Traditional health educators can have only a relatively small impact on people during most of their lives.* Doctors, nurses, teachers and community workers are usually the people we define as carrying out and providing the model of health education. But most people do not meet these professions during most of their health career. Outside of birth, old age and child-birth and care, those meetings that do occur are rare, very specific and of short duration.

It seems to be that the influence of these professionals and experts has decreased, a reduction concomitant with the rise of self-care and self-help with its questioning of professionalism and expertise. This questioning is based on a concern about the mystification and dependency often seen to be fostered by élite professions.

3. *Health care services, in their organization and main theories of operation, do not support the promotion of good health.* In the UK the National Health Service is overwhelmingly biased towards providing hospital services. In such a climate, it is

difficult for health promotion services to compete for resources. It is also difficult to gain resources because of the stark contrast of the major models of action. The caring activities of health care services are on the whole directed by a professional medical mechanical model. A health promotion approach emphasises the whole person, mass change and the giving away of knowledge. The latter issue is of particular importance. Giving away knowledge and information about health issues is in conflict with most professions whose power and influence is gained through the restriction and mystification of knowledge and *not* through giving it away. It is also probably true that most health care services do not present an image to the public of organizations that are concerned with their managerial or organizational health.

4. *The cost of providing health promotion services in a traditional way would be outrageously expensive.* There are just too many people to provide a 'professional' and detailed health education service to all and, anyway, one might question its benefits! Billions of pounds are spent in the UK each year on providing health care services. This money reaches, in any genuine sense of the word, only a small proportion of the population each year. Governments already question the proportion of the funds spent on the health sector. Think then of the additional cost of providing a comprehensive health education service where the *whole* population needs to be involved each and every year.

Combined together these dilemmas either lead to an impasse or guide us to seek out radical solutions and new ways to organize and direct health promotion.

Beyond Professionalism

A starting point for overcoming these dilemmas is to move away from a professional approach. Health education has grown up with the dogma that the role of the health education officer is to support the educational activities of the doctor, nurse, health visitor, etc. As we have seen earlier, this is unlikely, for structural reasons, to get to much of the population with a holistic and changing message; changing, because our knowledge of what is health and how to improve it is developing all the time with research and increased understanding.

Another aspect of this approach is one of ownership. Working through professionals automatically seems to ascribe power over information to these various élite groups, for example, the production of health education leaflets. Our experience of many leaflets is that they seem to end when they get to the interesting bit, telling you to go and see your doctor instead of what you can do about, or the consequences of, a medical condition.

A new approach to health education would try to redress the balance. The health promoter would gain the high ground between knowledge and the public. The role then would be direct to the public on mass with the intention of providing accurate and facilitating information and other services.

Taking this stance has its dangers. Gaining power through the control of knowledge is very common and corrupting. Even in health education units it is possible to find examples of information leaflets being controlled and re-stricted in access: 'The only people that can use these leaflets are profesionals in their educational activities!' 'Information on maternity and child care can only be given to pregnant women (why shouldn't a woman or anyone who is not pregnant have access to this information?)!' Another example is the common proposition that people can only be educated if the educator has control of the whole process. Use of mass media approaches are disparaged because health educators are concerned that people may not make proper use of the information offered. Instead, 'real' approaches are seen as getting groups together and assisting people to put knowledge into practise: control of the process from beginning to end! Such approaches, of course, mean that they meet very few people from the intended target group and these are selected from those people who are joiners of groups and are prepared to be controlled by others.

This latter scenario is in contravention of the megatrends of instant information, self-care and -help and multiple options. To counter this profes-sionalizing pressure in health education requires a very explicit understanding of our role.

People involved in health promotion should be professional but they are *not* a profession. They should be good at the methods of offering the widest possible access to health skills, environments and information, e.g. profession-al in the sense of being good at their job rather than gaining power by controlling information. Health promoters cannot be a profession because they are the antithesis of a profession!

Mass Approaches

Offering health information and healthy choices direct to the public and on a large scale is one answer to the health promotion dilemmas. Our experience in Mersey has provided a number of lessons about a mass or *populist* approach, an approach which is very different from the traditional one.

With this style of health promotion we need to take *a wider definition of health*, one which reflects more accurately the experience of real people. People are not, we hope, a collection of sexually transmitted disease and heart disease risk factors. Most people, given an opportunity to think about it, are well aware that health is a complex phenomenon. They can easily observe that their mental state of well-being is influenced by, and influences, their physical condition. To adapt to this, health promotion has to change from *vertical programmes* – hypothermia campaigns, nutrition campaigns, exercise campaigns, etc. The more appropriate approach is the *horizontal programme*. An example of this is the Age Well Campaign of the Health Education Authority, which is an inte-grated programme for promoting the health and well-being of older people across all aspects of their lives.

Building on where people are at is another important issue, as it is partly about riding on trends. It is also about offering starting points (multiple options) so that people can start learning not only about a subject that suits their requirements, but at a level which suits their present position. The latter we call *open learning*. Open learning is a special type of *participation*, and it is a very necessary part of a mass programme. It means providing, on a large scale, learning environments through which people can *choose* to start at a point which suits their present state of development, knowledge, skills, emotional involvement, etc., and then embark on a journey which is under their control and provides them with their own unique experience – an experience which is unique to them and yet can be catered for within a mass programme.

The reason for open learning and the other factors outlined is to encourage people to join a journey of self-discovery. To do this people must be motivated. All the processes outlined are ways of gaining motivation – motivation to change, without having a detailed long-term professional 'style' relationship, without unacceptable cost and loss of control, and with choice and freedom. Fun and enjoyment are also highly motivating and part of this approach. Learning and the motivation to learn are greatly enhanced by making the process one which is attractive and enjoyable.

There are two main ways to gain change. One is to change the world and people adapt to fit the new circumstances, and the other is for people to want to – to be motivated to – change and to have the tools and facilities to do it. Both are major aspects of the practise of health promotion. The first relates to political, policy and environmental change, the second to the *populist approach*.

Populism – an example

An example of a populist approach is provided by the Mersey Travelling Health Fair Scheme. This health promotion scheme, which is about physical fitness and healthy life-styles, has been visited by 500,000 people in under 2 years. Everyone that visited the scheme, at the International Garden Festival in Liverpool (1984) or on five converted double-decker buses, had the opportunity to have a personalized test of their fitness, stamina, strength and suppleness and a test of their healthy life-style. Open learning was provided by the use of low-cost computers (Commodore 64s) with user-friendly branched programs.

The computers allowed us to deprofessionalize the Health Fair and still provide personalized relevant and tailored advice. Computers and computer programs allow you to take professional/scientific knowledge and make it available to anyone that can use a keyboard and watch a TV screen. This approach is very cheap compared with employing expensive doctors and nurses to do the education job. Computers can be made available to a mass audience – 20 per cent of our region's population visited the Travelling Health Fairs in less than 2 years, and this was only one scheme! They are cheap and getting cheaper all the time, they are under the user's control and they provide standardized and authoritative messages.

Control is an interesting issue – before we started, we were told that people would not trust computers with confidential and sensitive information about themselves. We found the exact opposite – people seemed very happy to trust an inanimate object, probably more so than many human beings. The fact that they determined what happened, i.e. what questions they answered using the keyboards themselves, meant that the whole process was under their control. If they lied they only lied to themselves, for no other person was involved, and the lies were represented in the computer printout that they received.

Once professional knowledge was released and put into the computers we could staff the scheme with ordinary people. Anyone could become involved in health promotion, for there was no need to employ highly trained people, except the *real* experts who advised our computer programmer. We found that the criteria for the appointment of staff was more their sociability, i.e. their ability to deal in a friendly and communicative way with our large flow of customers. Over time I think that we demonstrated that the combination of computers and 'ordinary' friendly people was more powerful and certainly more communicative than having the scheme staffed by doctors, nurses and health education officers. We now believe that a long period of health science education appears to put people out of touch with other people, and certainly puts a professional distance between them.

By following this path we had stumbled across the megatrend *high-tech*/high touch. It seemed almost automatic that once we started using computer education on a large scale we needed to balance this with human contact. The young, previously unemployed Liverpudlians that manned the Health Fairs were the real stars of the show. Not only had we deprofessionalized health promotion with this populist approach but we had also opened up a previously untapped resource – the humour and human skills for which Liverpool is, or should be, renowned.

The staff put people at their ease and added their own ingredient of humour, making for a *fun* rather than a serious approach. They managed the flow of people through the Fairs, and performed fitness tests, the results of which were calculated by computer and each client received a personal and unique computer printout with a prescription for change. The staff helped people to interpret the printouts, not from the point of view of an expert but as an equal.

This populist approach allowed us to start with people on a journey of learning, beginning at a point of interest to them. They could then develop the *interaction* and take it further under their own control. The computers allow a considerable degree of self-controlled interaction, for it really only depends on the sophistication of the software, the programs and the state of knowledge. The starting point or topics of initial interest for a populist approach of this type are really a matter of judgement or gut feeling. They are closely linked with the concept of megatrends. One should choose a topic in which there is a growing interest, one which grabs people, e.g. 'I'd like to know how fit I am, how long I will live, etc.' One interesting point is that before we started, the Fairs' many professionals told us that ordinary people would not be interested in how fit they are or in having their life-style and stress level measured.

However, this was shown not to be the case. Apart from those people who visited the Fairs, a number of community groups in under-privileged areas contacted us and asked if we could make the Fairs mobile and bring them to their area. They usually said they had heard of the scheme from someone who had visited the International Garden Festival and had really enjoyed the Health Fair experience, and that people in their area couldn't afford the cost of the journey to the Fair.

Interaction is another element of participation, for to be actively involved in your own education is a well-known and powerful educational principle. Both using the computer keyboards and testing your own body through the fitness testing that was offered appealed to people and they seemed to gain more change than might usually be expected.

One less expected aspect of the Health Fairs was their multisectoral and commercial potential. Because they were large scale and popular they offered considerable opportunities for sponsorship and the involvement of organizations not usually connected with the health world. This led us to develop the idea of *self-sustaining health promotion*.

Self-sustaining Health Promotion

If you put together populist health promotion and multisectoral activity then you end up with some very interesting possibilities for the way that you can run health promotion programmes. Because of their popularity, populist activities can make self-sustaining if not profitable operations. Again this suggests one of the answers to the last of our initial dilemmas, i.e. the question of the cost of going out to meet very large numbers of people on a regular basis. *Body Mind Magic* provides the example of this style of operation.

Body Mind Magic

Body Mind Magic is a direct descendant of the Travelling Health Fairs. This proposed development is a cross between a Disney-style theme park and a science museum. It is the logical extension of the health fairs. It asks the question: 'How many things are there about me about how I work and my potential that could be explained through participative experiential exhibits?' It takes the concepts of the science centre and turns them on their head. Often in science centres we are the exhibit – our hearing and our eyesight are tested and then used to help us gain an understanding of scientific principles. Body Mind Magic takes the opposite approach. It uses science, technology, art and entertainment to explain us to ourselves. It uses computers, high tech, medical equipment and Disney-style presentations to allow people to find out about their bodies and minds. It is a populist way of unlocking for a mass audience the specialized knowledge of medicine, biology and psychology.

In terms of health promotion it operates on the basis that a keystone of health is that people should have an understanding of the way they work, not only at an intellectual but also at an emotional level. Body Mind Magic is an example of self-sustaining health promotion because it is not only a health promotion activity but it can also be seen as a tourist and cultural activity, an economic generator in its own right. It is being planned by a health promotion unit in a Health Authority but it is being taken forward by a Local Development Corporation and would, in the longer term, be run as a commercially-sponsored activity. It is predicted that it would attract more than 500,000 visitors a year and would become a major focus for populist health promotion.

Synthesis

The development of the plans for Body Mind Magic demonstrates all the processes outlined and can act to resolve the dilemmas. It takes a holistic view of health, and it is truly multisectoral, drawing on a wide range of scientific and artistic expertise. It would be born out of a Development Corporation and a Health Authority, and it would have been facilitated by the social entrepreneurial zeal of the members of a Health Promotion Unit and a wide network of associates. It is a horizontal programme taking as its starting point people's interest in themselves. It is a mass phenomenon drawing an audience to an event that is fun and provides an open learning experience. A major tenet of the experience is that it is participative and unique to every visitor.

6 Healthy Public Policy for the New Public Health

Virchow's conclusion that politics is medicine on a large scale underpins much of the debate which surrounds the New Public Health.[1] While there appears to be a broad measure of agreement across the political spectrum of the need for a new approach, that agreement breaks down when it comes to identifying the policies which are needed to support its development. Dimensions which are relevant in this debate include the victim-blaming versus structuralist and, to some extent, its counterpart the minimalist versus maximalist view of the role of the State. However, what is of particular interest about the new as opposed to the old public health is the extent to which libertarians of the left and right as opposed to authoritarians and paternalists may find themselves in the same camp on particular issues, e.g. compulsory testing for high-risk groups for AIDS, women's right to choose in relation to abortion, or the necessity for agricultural policies which promote good nutrition. The new social paradigm seems to cut across the old economic one.[2,3] The building of healthy public policies which are enabling, and which create supportive environments and strengthen community action on the basis of developed personal skills and health advocacy, challenges basic assumptions about the level of autonomy which individuals have a right to expect and about the extent to which corporate and State intervention is appropriate to ensure that autonomy.[4]

One aspect of this argument is the extent to which individuals have the right to take risks which might endanger their own or other people's health and the extent to which society accepts an obligation to provide for risk-takers and create a harm-reducing context for their behaviour. This arises particularly, for instance, where behaviours associated with the pursuit of sexual or drug-induced pleasure may be surrounded by moral condemnation from those holding particularly strong religious or moral views.

The idea of 'healthy public policy' is particularly associated with the work of Milio in the United States and Draper and his Unit for the Study of Health Policy in the United Kingdom.[5-7] The concept is, however, implicit in Lalonde's idea of the need to change the health field, the field in which health choices are influenced and formed, and is spelled out by Sigerist in his 'health programme for every country'.[8]

This need was made explicit in the United Kingdom in the Beveridge Report of 1942, which represented a consensus brought about by the appalling effects of the recession of the 1930s.[9] In the past, health policies were often manifested by specific public health and allied legislation and the establishment of specific health and social service organizations in many countries.

Milio has described a model which places health and the human organism in its complex biophysical and socio-economic environment (Fig. 6.1.) In this essentially ecological scheme human beings are part of a closed system where behaviours and environments are constantly interacting and where policies may be adopted which act at any of a large number of points. To optimize this effect it may well be necessary to have policies which act at a number of points. An agreed aim may be to optimize the positive options and minimize the negative ones, working to make healthy choices the easy choices.[5]

According to Milio:[5]

> Typical personal behaviour among Americans, even as variations occur is closely linked to a growth-orientated, industrial economy. It is a reflection at the personal level of directions taken on the national scale. The lavish use of energy for production brings more sedentary jobs and modes for transportation which reduce physical exercise and caloric expenditure. In order to obtain and retain what this affluent society makes available only to some, Americans have embraced a system of competition which requires time-orientated activity, calculation and fast pace which in turn contribute to accidents and generate distress. The ensuing desire to seek relief quickly makes for greater use of readily available 'solutions' such as cigarettes, alcohol and tranquilizers. Production for commercial consumption, valuing saleability first inevitably contributes to a reduction in the quality and safety of ambient air and water, of workplaces and of foods and other goods.
>
> At the same time that economic fluctuations change personal economic resources and modify consumption patterns, the web of social ties is itself changed. This stems from economy-based distress in families, resulting in more separations and divorce and from intensity of work place, loss of job security, consequent worker alienation, and diminishing labour organisational ties. All affect the pervasiveness of distress and the capacity of large proportions of the population to use effective coping patterns.

What is particularly disturbing is the scale of the modern public health disaster. In Victorian Europe appalling social, work and environmental conditions were created but they were essentially on a local basis, albeit with distant manifestations as a result of colonialism. In the multinational global village of today the problems are coalescing on an enormous scale, as is so

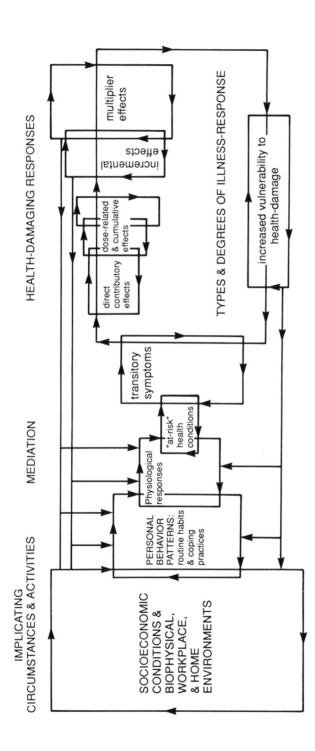

Fig. 6.1. Mutual-causal interconnections in contemporary health and illness.[5]

vividly demonstrated by the Chernobyl nuclear disaster in 1986, the European acid rain problem, and the ecological disasters represented by pollution of the Rhine, the clearance of the Amazon basin and destruction of the remaining world commons as well as the disappearance of the ozone layer. All in all we are doing a poor job as 'Stewards of the Earth' for future generations.[10–13]

Writers such as Robertson and McKnight have spelled out the needs for a new paradigm, a *Sane* alternative which respects human and social integrity and that of the world's environment as part of a strategy for social and economic regeneration based on the empowerment of the population:[15,16] in Robertson's words, SHE (Sane, Humane and Ecological) rather than HE (Hyper-expansionist). Such an approach is likely to include an appraisal of community resources and skills as well as of needs and a focus on how resources and skills may be enhanced and liberated to promote the public health.[17] A reduction in the power of professions and in the induced dependency of individuals and communities on them is likely to be part of that process.

Levels of Policy and Action

Systematic action to improve public health requires simultaneous action on a broad front and at different levels (Fig. 6.2.). The inadequacy of the narrow victim-blaming approach must be apparent if one considers for example the macro-environmental issues. Action to prevent a recurrence of the Chernobyl disaster requires international governmental policies and collaboration. Even familiar problems such as the prevention of coronary heart disease and the curbing of tobacco consumption go much wider and higher than traditional health education about risk factors. There is a need to address issues such as the deliberate creation of ill-health and the exporting of health problems to the third world by the marketing of health-damaging products. In fact, three types of health education for public health have been described as necessary if public health really is to involve the public:[6]

1. *Biological knowledge*: the nuts and bolts about how our bodies and relationships work and how to promote and maintain them.
2. *Consumer information*: about the services which are available to help us to improve and maintain our health (how to get the best out of the system, what is available and how to complain when necessary).
3. *The big issues which affect health*: unemployment, schooling, agriculture, pollution of the air, water and food, road traffic and public transport, exploitation of the world's ecology and the global commons. The activities of the anti-health sector of the economy.[18]

Usually when people talk about health education it is only type 1 which is included. All governments and statutory agencies tend to be apprehensive about types 2 and 3, because an informed public makes demands, seeks to share control and will challenge vested interests. This is exactly what the New Public Health is about.

LEVEL OF ACTION	HEALTH PROMOTION	PREVENTION		
		PRIMARY	SECONDARY	TERTIARY
INTERNATIONAL, NATIONAL, LOCAL GOVERNMENT				
INSTITUTIONAL				
PERSONAL				

HEALTH EDUCATION

Fig. 6.2.   Levels of action for the New Public Health.

Even type 1 education is not unproblematical – that people should be in possession of the factual information necessary to make informed health choices. Conflict over exactly what may be taught about sexuality in school systems and who may decide course content is common. Until the prevention of AIDS became an imperative, the promotion of condoms to teenagers to prevent unwanted pregnancy as well as sexually transmitted diseases was impossible in many places because of the objection of adults who would wish to try and control teenagers' sexual autonomy.

The Elements of Healthy Public Policy: Information, Advocacy, Intervention, Evaluation

INFORMATION

The power of information is often alluded to in public health and the tradition of the use of statistics to influence health policy goes back at least as far as Graunt (in the United Kingdom).[19] Duncan demonstrated just how effective descriptive local health data can be with his report on the high rate of mortality in Liverpool. Duncan's report, lectures and pamphlet played an important part in making the case for Medical Officers of Health; they also provided information which was drawn on in drafting the first English Public Health Act of 1848 and helped to establish the precedent of the annual reports produced by Medical Officers of Health until 1974.[20,21]

The importance of this aspect of Duncan's work is in his instinctive recognition of the power of local data. People do not accept statistics as having relevance unless they have immediacy and concern themselves or their own community. It is said that there is no good or bad except by comparison; if that comparison can harness some of the competitive instincts which characterize any community it is likely to be all the more energizing in its effects. Competition between British cities to reduce mortality rates was certainly a motivating factor in the nineteenth century.

Recent examples of the motivating power of comparative data include the *Seven Countries Heart Disease Study* whose findings stimulated the Karelia Project for the community control of heart disease (Table 6.1),[22] and the galvanizing effect which the publication of an international comparison of teenage pregnancy in 37 developed countries appears to have had on policy initiatives in the United States.[23]

The study found a teenage pregnancy rate of 96 per 1000 15–19 year olds per annum in the United States compared with 45 in England and Wales, 35 in Sweden and 14 in the Netherlands, against a background of similar levels of sexual activity; one particular policy initiative which it has led to in many States has been the introduction of high-school-based birth control advisory centres.

The whole genre of reports on inequalities in health is in the same tradition of health data being made available and informing debate about policy options. In the case of the Black Report on inequalities in health in Britain it has been followed by a succession of such reports with an increasing focus on inequalities at the local level.[24,25]

In the same way that individuals are more open to change at some times in their lives than others, e.g. stopping smoking if given anti-smoking informa-

Table 6.1   The Seven Countries Heart Disease Study
(WHO Collaborative Study of Myocardial Infarction, 1971)

Helsinki	7.4
Nijmegen	4.8
Perth	4.6
London	4.3
Heidelberg Kaunas (USSR) Berlin	2.6
Sofia	1.7

Rates per 1000 men aged 20–64 years.

---

* The Karelia Question, – who was it who asked for the comparative data on heart disease death rates and thereby set the agenda? Was it the people themselves or their medical advisers? Ideally, the questions should come from an informed public but it is a chicken and egg situation – who informs the public? How can a non-paternalistic balance be struck?

tion when they have a smoking-related illness episode, communities are more likely to be receptive to some information, depending on how and when it is presented and on whether the request for information has come from the community itself.*

It follows that communities may not give the same priority to the same information as professionals would. Nor must it be assumed that the only valid data is of a quantitative, statistical kind. Anthropological and sociological perspectives are most valuable in making explicit other more subtle perspectives – oral histories and photographic records may turn out to be powerful tools for change in public health (Fig. 6.3).

There are important implications for the training and style of work of professionals in public health, including primary medical care. There is a particular need for a new kind of field epidemiology which respects person- and community-centred views.[26–30] This is one area where there is a potential for creating new jobs of value to the community, i.e. as health information officers.

Case Study: Shopping and Coronary Prevention in Liverpool
Heart disease and stroke between them account for one-third of deaths before the age of 75 in the Mersey Region. Within the region, the Liverpool Health District experiences some of the highest death rates to be found in any district and the rates for heart disease and stroke are 20–30 per cent higher than those for England as a whole.[32]

Factors which are known to be associated with increased risk of death from these diseases include:

● excessive consumption of alcohol,
● lack of exercise,
● stress,
● smoking,
● obesity.

They also include specific nutritional factors; in particular, diets which have a high fat content (especially saturated fat), are high in refined sugar and salt and are low in fibre.

In 1983, the National Advisory Committee on Nutrition Education (NACNE) recommended changes in six areas of diet as part of a strategy to reduce ill-health from heart disease and other conditions associated with dietary factors:[33]

1. Reduction in total fat consumption and reduction in saturated fat consumption aided by introducing polyunsaturates as an alternative.
2. Reduction in sugar intake.
3. Reduction in salt intake.
4. Reduction in alcohol consumption.
5. Increase in dietary fibre.
6. To maintain the energy value of food, but to shift from current sources to low-fat foods, bread, fruit and vegetables.

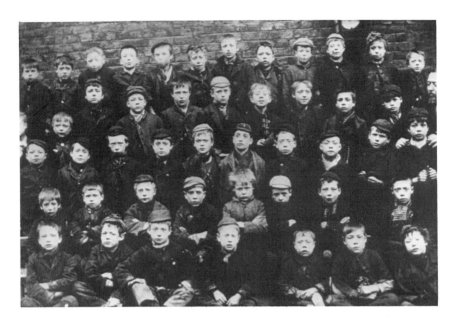

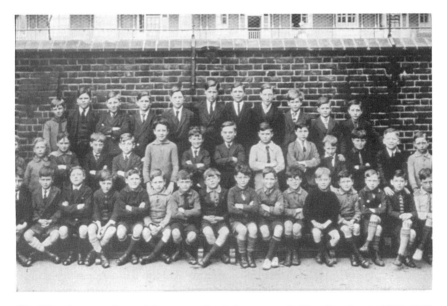

Fig. 6.3.   A comparison of the same school class group in East London in 1900, 1925 and 1950. These photographs constitute powerful comparative data, demonstrating as they do the improvements in growth, development and health during this period, largely as a result of policies outside the medical sector. (With acknowledgement to the late Sidney Chave.)

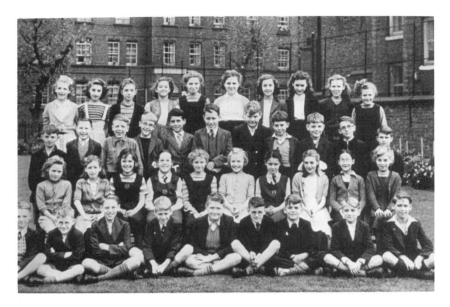

Fig. 6.3   (contd.)

The report recommended that health education should be channelled towards these aims.

The coronary prevention group, in launching its initiative for action to prevent heart disease in 1984, incorporated the NACNE recommendations into its objectives to be set for Health Authorities and, most recently, the Committee on Medical Aspects of Food Policy (COMA) has endorsed what are essentially the same recommendations.[34,35] In view of this emerging consensus on the risk factors involved and the need to change them, it was felt that more information was needed to clarify the extent and distribution of risk factors in the Liverpool population.

In order to obtain further information a survey was carried out to ascertain the attitudes and knowledge of people in five areas of Liverpool towards food and towards their own eating habits and tobacco consumption.[36] The study was based on interviews with 100 people from each of five areas. Four of these areas are in the inner city and tend to be characterized by high unemployment, a low proportion of owner-occupiers and a number of other indicators of social and material disadvantage. A recent analysis has shown that they also have the highest death rates in the city, including premature deaths from heart disease. The fifth area was chosen for comparison because it is an affluent part of the city with no apparent indications of deprivation or poor health.[25,37]

Representative samples were interviewed from each area as they left their local supermarket by asking them questions about their diet and shopping habits, particularly focussing on the known risk factors.

Although this was a pilot study, a consistent picture emerged which was compatible with the mortality patterns of the areas concerned. It was found that those people living in the favoured area of the city were much further along the road to having implemented the NACNE and Coronary Prevention Group recommendations for themselves and their families than people from the deprived inner-city areas or the post-war public housing estate included in the survey. The former shopper profile could be described as 'salt-conscious, high-fibre, low-fat, non-smoking' as compared with the latter profile of 'salt-adding, low-fibre, high-fat and smoking'.

Faced with these findings one might be tempted to go along with those who suggest that the solution to people's health problems lies with themselves and that they should change their behaviour. That such a victim-blaming conclusion is simplistic and based on an incomplete understanding of the situation is made clear from a consideration of the problem, bearing in mind the Ottawa Charter as a framework.[38]

The food which people eat is at the end of a chain of production, distribution and marketing. What people buy for their families and themselves depends on their income, knowledge, motivation and skills and what is available. During the period of the survey one of the researchers made a point of doing his own family's shopping at each of the supermarkets in turn which were under study. It became readily apparent that, even if you knew what you should be doing, for many people the exercise of healthy choice was not possible for the following reasons. First, healthy food tends to be more expensive than unhealthy food. People who are on low incomes have as their main priority the prevention of hunger and to make their money spin out until the next Social Security cheque.

Second, in parts of Liverpool, 90 per cent of households do not have access to a private motor car and, therefore, these families are restricted in their shopping choice to whatever is locally available. This has been reinforced by the deterioration in public transport services since the deregulation of the buses. In many of the poorer parts of the city, people may not even have access any longer to a down-market supermarket, but to a high-priced corner shop or mobile shop selling predominantly processed and tinned rather than fresh food.

This situation is further exacerbated by the granting of planning approval for large, edge-of-town hypermarkets, catering for the mobile, wage-earning middle-classes. Developments such as these lead to a knock-on effect of closures of stores in other areas, further restricting the choice of those who are not mobile in favour of those who are. The prevention of this kind of insidious erosion of choice needs support in the structure plan for cities through explicit planning policy. It may also need financial support for local shops as has happened in parts of Denmark.

A third reason is food labelling. Knowledge of NACNE or COMA alone is insufficient to enable the discerning shopper to buy healthy food because of the poor labelling in many retail outlets.

A Lack of Skills
There are gaps in knowledge and many people no longer have the skills to

prepare fresh food or cheap alternatives to convenience food. In part, there appears to have been a 'deskilling' of a whole generation as a result of the promotion and success of convenience foods. Again there is a danger of seeing this in simplistic victim-blaming terms. One·of the main reasons for the demand for convenience food, possibly beginning with breast-milk substitute, was the benefit to women who frequently worked outside the home and then were expected to produce a family meal at the end of a working day. The answer to convenience food is not to do away with it but, on the one hand, to improve its quality and, on the other, to provide education and training to both boys and girls of all intellectual abilities from an early age in domestic science and cooking in order that the work may be shared in adult life and the need for convenience foods be reduced.

Similarly, junk-food restaurants serve a very important social function – that of enabling people on low incomes to eat out; an important part of life which is perhaps too readily taken for granted by health education professionals who are able to afford healthier eating places. What is needed is better-quality, cheap restaurants, not their abolition.

Obtaining this kind of information is the first step to developing policies appropriate to the problem. The way in which that information is then used highlights the importance of effective health advocacy. Clearly, supportive policies for coronary prevention need to be wide-ranging and incorporate, among other things income maintenance, town planning, agricultural and transport policy, food labelling and education, and have local, national and international dimensions.

HEALTH ADVOCACY

The relative autonomy and protected position of the British Medical Officer of Health, and his (they were, apparently, all male) freedom to represent the health interests of his public at least until 1974, is a touchstone for those seeking to develop health advocacy. There are few satisfactory models around today and it is easier to blame the victim than to indict powerful organized groups or commercial interests which are working against the public health.

The civic administration in Toronto has continued to be structured on the old British model and the public health department has an advocacy section which has pursued issues relating to poverty, unemployment, food and energy. In contrast, in the United Kingdom, the post-1974 community physician is seen very much as a civil servant who should stay out of controversy. When a Bill to enforce the use of seat-belts in cars was before Parliament in 1982, those community physicians who wrote to the members of parliament in their areas and asked them to support the legislation were reprimanded. More recently, one community physician has been suspended for advocating the installation of condom vending machines in high schools and another for criticizing her employing authority for making cost-saving cuts in the family planning services.

The same constraint has not been in evidence with regard to the views of senior police officers, and the Chief Constable of Manchester has become well known for his views on the morality of a homosexual life-style and the appropriate ways in which to treat criminals. It might seem reasonable for the defenders of the public health to have at least as great a freedom of expression as the members of the police constabulary! This problem seems to be common to many countries with administrations of differing political persuasion.

The first level of advocacy is the actual generation of descriptive and analytical information. The second lies in its being made available in an accessible form to the general public, opinion formers and policy makers and being represented with the authority of technical competence. Clearly, a close working relationship with the media is essential at this stage.

Within the Mersey Region the Liverpool University Department of Community Health has been able to play a useful role as, for example, in providing a public forum with expert input to debate the implications of the recurrent episodes of the public water supply. However, the limitations on developing health advocacy from a government-controlled health authority base became apparent over issues surrounding challenges to the marketing practices of the tobacco industry – it proved difficult to agree the wording for a press release responding to the test marketing of tobacco chewing pouches in the region (a region with sufficient health problems without adding cancer of the buccal cavity), and controversial when the Regional Health Promotion Unit publicly distanced itself from a street festival with tobacco sponsorship.

One example where very targeted advocacy seems to have been effective, was in relation to the tardiness of milk distributors in the region in responding to consumer demands for doorstep deliveries of fresh skimmed milk. As a letter to the editor of *Community Medicine* states:

> When I returned to this area almost two years ago, one of the first things I did was to try and order a doorstep delivery of fresh, skimmed milk. After several failures, I decided to go to the top. I first phoned the marketing manager of probably the largest retailer and asked him why it was not possible to obtain fresh skimmed milk from his milkman in Liverpool, whilst it had been in Southampton – I was told that there was no demand for it in Liverpool. My response was to tell him that I thought he should take steps to supply it as, if I had anything to do with it, there would soon be a demand as a result of health promotional activities within the region.
>
> The next dairy that I tried said that yes, they did supply fresh skimmed milk, so I placed an order. The following day the milkman left UHT (sterilised skimmed milk) on the doorstep – the Company didn't actually know what they were selling.
>
> We put up with the UHT for many months until one evening there was an article in the local paper telling Liverpool women to order fresh skimmed milk to protect their husband's hearts – the article claimed that

the product was freely available on the doorstep. At this point, I wrote a letter to the paper disputing the statement and I was promptly taken to task by the marketing manager who I had spoken to 12 months before – fresh skimmed milk was freely available, he said, and had been for some time – clearly he had acted on my advice.

Within days, our own milkman mysteriously substituted fresh skim for the UHT. A bit paranoid by now, I phoned the depot manager to find out what was happening. He told me that he had no idea but that a few days previously he had been told by his boss to find some fresh skimmed milk from anywhere and make it available. He had bought it in from Cheshire and it was going very well!

Curious, I sent a short questionnaire to all 97 dairies listed in the Merseyside and Cheshire Yellow Pages. Information was provided very promptly by 42 (43 per cent). Of these, 38 were supplying fresh skimmed milk on the doorstep – 26 of them having commenced to supply it within the previous 6 months.

Many dairies had also begun to supply other low fat products.

The reasons given for the changes in product availability centred on consumer demand and on the effects of recent television programmes on public opinion. I would like to think that my own intervention gave the movement to skimmed milk a shove in the right direction, because the Company I had contacted is one of six which have the market almost sewn up between them. The rapid response of a second of the six reflects the competition which currently exists in milk marketing and gives an indication of the commercial advantages open to those alert enough to the growing demand for healthier products.

J.A. 1984.

In areas such as the north of England the need for effective health advocacy on behalf of the poor, the inadequately housed, the unemployed and disadvantaged has never been greater. The polarization of wealth and power is being accelerated deliberately as part of government policy and the middle-classes have failed to take advantage of their limited opportunities to demonstrate solidarity with the dispossessed.

INTERVENTION

Short-life Working Groups (Top-down)
Public health practitioners and academics have opportunities to initiate or support interventions both from within and outside their host organizations: the production of a community diagnosis and the use of it to help set a new health agenda is one example, participation in short-life policy working groups is another. These groups seem to work best when they have clear terms of

reference, a limited time in which to report and a focus on identifying what is possible within the existing resources and arrangements. However, this approach of focussing on what is possible within the involved agencies can simultaneously be used to identify where action is needed at a higher level in support of local policy initiatives, perhaps nationally or internationally. Within Mersey, examples of short-life policy groups have included ones on nutrition, exercise and tranquillizer dependence.

Public bodies are frequently in a powerful position to influence policy not only within their own organizations, but within others at the same or a higher level, as well as by the effective advocacy of appropriate recommendations. For example, Robin Ireland who has responsibility for exercise promotion in the Mersey Region established a working party to recommend policy. The recommendations of the Mersey Exercise policy guidelines are as follows:

RECOMMENDATIONS
to District Health Authoritities and
Family Practitioner Committees

1. A formal exercise policy should be adopted to include the accompanying recommendations.
2. A health education/promotion officer or an identified person should be assigned to implement the policy.
3. The policy should be fully researched and evaluated.
4. The health benefits of regular physical exercise should be widely publicized, and information should be provided on safe levels of exercise according to age and level of physical fitness. The relationship between stress and positive health should be recognized as a part of the exercise policy.

Recommendations can be subdivided for implementation within the NHS.

(a) *on NHS premises*

5. Exercise facilities should be provided for use both by NHS staff and by patients. Changing and showering facilities should likewise be made available.
6. DHAs should actively support both administratively and financially the formation of clubs which are available to all NHS staff and which promote physical recreation activities.
7. Facilities should be provided to allow suitably trained people, such as Look After Yourself (LAY) tutors, to run exercise and stress-related programmes both for staff and patients.
8. DHAs should fund and allow time for NHS staff to train in appropriate skills such as LAY training.
9. Rehabilitation programmes for patients such as those with cardiac problems should be widely available.
10. Rehabilitation programmes should include advice on safe exercise and should set up networks between physiotherapy facilities and outpatient

departments on NHS premises and recreation facilities in the community.

11. There is a need for specialist Sports Injuries Clinics to promote rehabilitation and to encourage and maintain safe levels of participation.

(b) *the NHS and the community*

12. NHS primary health care staff should be enabled to run suitable programmes – such as LAY – in the community, and on non-NHS premises where necessary.

13. Contacts should be encouraged and networks set up between local recreation facilities and doctors' surgeries, health clinics and health centres. Relevant sports information should be made readily available and widely displayed.

14. GPs and other primary health care workers should be encouraged to make referrals to appropriate recreation agencies.

15. The needs of special interest groups such as the elderly and the disabled should be recognized, and exercise and relaxation facilities made available to all.

16. DHAs should promote exercise policies with local employers.

17. Exercise and recreational activities should be encouraged in all residential homes.

RECOMMENDATIONS
to Local Authorities

1. A formal exercise and health policy should be considered to include the accompanying recommendations.

2. The policy should be fully researched and evaluated.

3. The health benefits of regular physical exercise should be widely publicized, and information should be provided on safe levels of exercise according to age and level of physical sport.

Recommendations can be subdivided for implementation.

(a) *within Education Department*

4. A health education advisor should be appointed to advise on the implementation of the policy.

5. Teachers should be trained in health education issues.

6. Schools should include health education in the existing curriculum and make health issues more relevant to students' needs.

7. Physical education teachers should be aware both of the needs of the talented and less able students. Team and individual sports should allow both for competition and non-competitive participation.

8. Physical education teachers should promote alternative exercise activities, such as exercise to music, which are likely to be carried on after leaving school in order to establish a regular exercise habit.

9. School facilities should be dual use when possible and every attempt made to enable the community to use them.
10. The needs of girls, ethnic minorities, and the disabled should be considered in a true equal opportunities policy.

(b) *within departments with a responsibility for recreation*

11. A community development/liaison officer should be appointed to advise on the implementation of the policy.
12. Recreation staff should be trained in health issues and encouraged to train as Look After Yourself (LAY) tutors where appropriate.
13. Recreation staff should set up LAY classes and similar health-based programmes in order to attract non-participants into their centres.
14. Publicity and sessions should reflect the needs of all members of the community and not just those of the most active participants.
15. Information on exercise facilities should be available and displayed in local centres such as supermarkets and health centres.
16. Special concessionary charges should be considered to encourage non-participants.
17. Creches should be made available to enable the parents of young children to use facilities.
18. Sports centres should ensure participants and visitors are made aware of the health benefits of exercise as noted in (2).
19. If sports centres offer refreshment facilities, these should be in line with DHA current nutrition and alcohol policy wherever possible.

(c) *within Social Services departments*

20. An officer should be appointed to advise on the implementation of the policy.
21. Social services staff should be trained in health issues and encouraged to train as Look After Yourself (LAY) tutors where appropriate.
22. Exercise and active recreational activities should be promoted with residential homes, day centres, luncheon clubs, etc.
23. Premises owned by social services should be made available to the community where possible for recreational use.
24. Care should be taken to promote healthy exercise for special groups such as the elderly and the disabled.

RECOMMENDATIONS
for consideration by management and trade unions for
implementation in the workplace

1. The value of exercise should be recognized as a part of a healthier life-style.
2. Staff and members should be encouraged to take part in regular active physical exercise.
3. Exercise facilities should be provided where possible. Changing and

showering facilities should likewise be made available.
4. Staff clubs which promote physical recreation activities should be supported; these may consider post-retirement activities.
5. Rehabilitation programmes should be provided.
6. Staff and members who may be able to lead exercise-based sessions should be trained in appropriate skills such as Look After Yourself.
7. Links should be maintained with local exercise facilities, and special arrangements considered to use local authority and private premises.

RECOMMENDATIONS
on appropriate regular physical exercise

It is widely accepted that for general protective exercise, appropriate activity should be rhythmic and should be maintained for 20–30 minutes, 2–3 times a week. Such activities as those listed below are effective:

- brisk walking,
- jogging/running,
- skipping,
- disco dancing,
- cycling,
- swimming,
- bench stepping.

*   *   *

Other policies have been developed in relation to harm reduction for intravenous drug users and the prevention of AIDS in conjunction with standing committees of the public and professionals.

Building Policy from Below
The problem with building policy from above, quite apart from the philosophical objection to top-down approaches, is that it then has to be 'sold' to the people who have to apply it. For this reason the mixed Standing Committee of community activists, technocrats and politicians is preferable to a narrowly drawn technical group. The next step is for professionals to meet the public at street level and to work with them in the formation of policy and policy demands. A good example of this has been the collaboration between Mersey Regional Health Authority, Liverpool Housing Trust, Merseyside Improved Houses, the Centre for Employment Initiatives, Wilkinson Hindle Architects, Liverpool Polytechnic and University and various other agencies and individuals with the Eldon Street Community Association in Liverpool 3.

Eldon Street is situated in the Vauxhall ward of Liverpool, half a mile north of the city centre in the heart of Liverpool's dockland.[12] The Community in this area is largely descended from the Irish Catholics who came to Liverpool as refugees during the potato famine of 1848 and afterwards. Until comparatively recently, it has been an area of remarkably high-density slum housing, there being seven parishes with all parish functions in the one ward. During the early part of the century many of the slum courts were demolished and the first council houses in the country were built.

During the 1960s a great deal more housing was cleared and thousands of families were moved to live on the new overspill estates at the edge of the city. Friends and neighbours were split up and social networks were destroyed. The disruption is widely held by local people to have led to the premature death of many elderly people. In 1978, when the city council decided without consultation that it was time to demolish the remaining slums, the community resisted. The Eldon Street Community Association (its motto was 'we do it better together') was formed with a street-based committee structure and the local people set about fighting for the right to be rehoused locally. They conducted their own surveys of people's housing wishes and embarked on a long struggle to build housing cooperatives.

In 1982 this community, which was already greatly stressed, received a body blow when the Tate and Lyle sugar refinery, the major local employer, closed with the loss of 2000 jobs. Thousands of other jobs in port-related work were lost within the space of several years and the adult male unemployment rate rose above 50 per cent.

We know that unsatisfactory housing can adversely affect health in a variety of ways.[43,44] We are also now aware of the strong and significant associations between unemployment and both mental and physical ill-health. In the case of mental illness, the causal nature of these associations has been established beyond doubt. The range of mental health problems identified includes depression, para-suicide and suicide itself.[45-47] As with physical health, the incidence of problems increases with the duration of unemployment. The range of physical disorders includes heart disease, chronic bronchitis, lung cancer and infant growth retardation.

In Vauxhall, housing, environmental, economic and social stress converge to produce the worst health in Liverpool: standardized mortality ratios 50 per cent higher than those for England and Wales; more than two-thirds of the school children in receipt of free school meals; a ratio of 1 in 200 school leavers going on to further education compared with 1 in 5 in the affluent ward of Woolton – all of these give an indication of the enormity of the problem. For the community itself its priority has been housing and then jobs. The community has had a strong belief in the importance of a sense of place in their own well-being, an understanding which is only now beginning to be taken seriously by academics.[48]

After 10 years of struggle the Community Association has now built the largest housing cooperative in the country, is in the process of establishing a range of community businesses, including some based on the potential of healthy products, and has developed the functions of its strong social networks to provide social care for the elderly and, for instance, ensuring that entitlements to surplus food from the European Common Market are fully taken up. The community now looks at buildings and derelict land within its area as unused resources and is actively seeking ways of bringing them into use, both socially and economically, as sports centres, workshops for community-owned businesses or recreation areas.

Questions have begun to be asked about the quality of medical services in the area, and expectations have been raised. The Eldonians have set a new style for working with professionals in which the professionals are seen to be 'on tap not on top'. It has been a two-way learning process, which recognizes McKnight's criticism of welfare programmes in which a majority of budgets benefits professionals rather than the poor.[16]

People with no formal education after they left school at the minimum school leaving age now have a strong and increasing sense of their power, of their rights and of their possibilities; professionals who have become involved with them had the satisfaction of working in a new, democratic and participative way. In the medium- to long-term there is little doubt that what is happening in Vauxhall will lead to improved physical, mental and social well-being.

What it has meant in practice for professionals working with the Eldonians has been that they have had to be willing to respond to requests for knowledge, information, skills, access to networks and resources as facilitators. It has meant, for instance, the Regional Health Authority Treasurers Department acting as banker for the establishment of an urban horticultural centre, and the University botanical nurseries acting as host to unemployed Eldonians being trained in cultivation methods by the staff of the Lancashire County Agricultural College. The Liverpool Housing Trust, whose mainstream work has been to provide high-quality low-rental homes to those on low income, has become involved in many ways, using its resources and its infrastructure in support of the Eldonians' plans. A major commercial food company has also become involved in the support of management development of community-owned business. It has challenged the housing and environment policies of government and changed the way in which people think about health.*

EVALUATION

The evaluation of interventions as comprehensive as that which is being pursued by the Eldon Street Community Association is not easy. On one level, the major questions are about reducing the inequalities of mortality and disease between Vauxhall and the favoured parts of Liverpool and the country as a whole; such outcomes, if they are achieved, will take a generation or more.

---

* There is a story about an agency in Asia going into a village with a very high infant mortality rate from gastroenteritis and diarrhoeal disease and constructing latrines without consulting the village leaders as to their own priorities. On returning 2 years later, they found the latrines unused. At this point the community was consulted and it was found that their priority was the elephants. Every year the elephants would trample down the sugar just when it was nearly ripe and the village was losing a major part of its potential income. The agency now cooperated with the villagers in finding ways to keep the elephants out. Later they began to discuss sanitation.

Yet most academic approaches to evaluation are limited to a time scale of several years and focus on specific cause and effect relationships; the germ model of disease and the magic bullet solution of an antibiotic or surgical intervention continues to dominate scientific thought. Within health service systems there is a strong emphasis on value for money and on measures of efficiency – effectiveness is rarely addressed.[49]

Even in recent large-scale public health interventions such as the Karelia Project and Heartbeat Wales, where changes in processes involving intervening variables in relation to risk factors have been included, it is difficult to claim credit for an intervention in achieving an effect against a backcloth of massive trends in more healthful behaviour.[22,50]

So far, there has been little effort made to address the fundamental evaluation issue raised by the New Public Health – if public health is people-centred, in keeping with the spirit of Health for All and the Ottawa Charter, not only must people themselves define their own health problems but they must also be central to any assessment of whether an intervention is worthwhile. Five strands appear to be necessary for evaluation research.

1. *The need for positive indicators in place of negative ones and for qualitative and small area data.* Most data that is currently available for the 12 health promotion priorities in the Mersey Region is medical/pathological or administrative in nature, whereas health promotion needs to focus on the healthy rather than the sick and on processes rather than on organization. Such data is difficult to relate to 'community' denominators; there is a particular deficiency of special survey data at small area level and of 'soft' descriptive data at any level.

Indicators of participation and intersectoral function do not currently exist and those of networking, empowerment and community morale are illustrative of others which need to be developed.

2. *The need to focus on contexts as well as people.* The necessity to avoid victim-blaming and to address the issue of contexts which support healthy choice in life-styles is well-illustrated by the problem of coronary prevention and shopping in Liverpool.[36] Clearly, among the mesh of factors – knowledge and attitudes, income, geography, transport – retail choice is the real focus for research in this area.

3. *Doing things from where people are.* People- and community-centred research is necessary. The traditional model of public health was a paternalistic one. Having identified hazards to the public health, the Medical Officer of Health had access to the whole panoply of public health legislation with which to enforce his recommended action. In turn this has led to a tendency with the New Public Health to attempt to travel the same route. Prescription based on epidemiological analysis tends to be the logical outcome of medically-based health promotion programmes. Such programmes tend to be top-down rather than bottom-up and vertical rather than horizontal.

Vertical programmes such as specific coronary prevention initiatives impose a disease-based model on everyday life and life-styles. The alternative is to provide support for processes which integrate different aspects of a healthy life-style at the community level, but which start from everybody's own interest in their own health, and that of their family and their social group, the organizational counterpart being primary care.

4. *The need for true stories.* Above all we need true stories of what really happened when somebody or a group of people tried to do something: John Snow and the Broad Street pump, Karelia and Stanford, the Welsh Heart Project and the Liverpool Project on teenage pregnancy. These are folk stories of public health and the parables for training new generations of workers, yet what was the truth in each case? Who did what, when and why? Really? Did the initiative really come from the 'community' or were professionals involved in a softening up process first? Did they give history a shove? Why was this project funded now, but not a similar project sooner or later or a project on a different topic but with a similar methodology? So we really do need true stories – yet if we had really known the truth, would the inspiration provided by some of the myths have led to real achievements?

5. *Assessment of the health promoting capabilities of a community.* It seems likely that the prerequisite for effective community participation in health promotion includes the availability of accurate information and the possibility of remedial action at the right time and in the right place – how were these conditions created? We need to find ways in which to describe communities which take account of community improvement and self-esteem, the collective and social equivalents of concepts which we understand well for the individual. Erikson's developmental approach to the tasks of maturation seems pertinent here as does the whole field of work on locus of control.[52,54]

References

1. Virchow, R.L.K. (1848). *Die Medizinische Reform*, p.2. Quoted in Sigerist, H.E. (1941). *Medicine and Human Welfare*, p. 93. Yale University Press, New Haven.
2. Labonte, R. and Penfold, S. (1981). Canadian perspectives in health promotion – a critique. *Health Education* April, 4–9.
3. Doyal, L. (1981). *The Political Economy of Health*. Pluto Press, London.
4. World Health Organization, Health and Welfare, Canada and Canadian Public Health Association (1986). Ottawa Charter For Health Promotion. *Canadian Journal of Public Health* 77 (6), 425–30.
5. Milio, N. (1986). *Promoting Health Through Public Policy*. Canadian Public Health Association, Ottawa, Canada.
6. Dennis, J., Draper, P., Griffiths, J., Partridge, J., Popay, J. and others (1979). *Rethinking Community Medicine. Unit for the Study of Health Policy.* Guy's Hospital, London.
7. St. George, D. and Draper, P. (1981). A health policy for Europe. *Lancet* ii, 463–5.
8. Sigerist, H. (1941). *Medicine and Human Welfare*. Oxford University Press, Oxford.
9. Beveridge, W. (1942). *The Social Insurance and Allied Services*. HMSO, London.
10. Bruntland, G.H. (1987). *Our Common Future. The World Commission on Environment and Development*. Oxford University Press, Oxford.
11. Myers, N. (ed.), (1985). *The Gaia Atlas of Planet Management*. Pan Books, London.
12. Barney, G.O. (1982). *The Global 2000 Report to the President: Entering the 21st Century*. Penguin, Harmondsworth.

13. Sampson, A. (ed.) (1980). *North–South. A Programme for Survival*. Pan Books, London.
14. Schumacher, E.E. (1974). *Small is Beautiful*. Sphere Books, London.
15. Robertson, J. (1985). *Future Work*. Gower/Temple, Smith, London.
16. McKnight, J.L. (1985). Regenerating Community. Paper presented to the Canadian Mental Health Associations Search Conference, Ottawa, 1985.
17. Rodale, R. (1987). *Regeneration, Building Healthy Communities*, Vol. 3, No. 5 Rodale Press, Emmaus, PA.
18. Player, D. (1987). The Fifth Duncan Memorial Lecture. University of Liverpool, Liverpool. *Public Health* **103** (4), 263–79.
19. Grant, J. (1662). *Natural and Political Observations made upon the Bills of Mortality, London*. Republished by Johns Hopkins Press, Baltimore, 1939.
20. Duncan, W.H., (1843). The physical causes of the high rate of mortality in Liverpool. Quoted in Fraser, W.M. (1947). *Duncan of Liverpool*. Hamish Hamilton, London.
21. Watkin, B. (1975). *Documents on Health and Social Services (1834), to the Present Day*. Methuen, London.
22. *Community Control of Cardiovascular Diseases. The North Karelia Project* (1981). Published on behalf of the National Public Health Laboratory of Finland by the WHO Regional Office for Europe.
23. Jones, E.F., Forrest, J.D., Goldman, N., Henshaw, S.K., Lincoln, R., Rosoff, J.S., Westoff, C.F. and Wulf, D. (1985). Teenage pregnancy in developed countries: determinants and policy implications. *Family Planning Perspectives* **7** (2), 53–63.
24. Townsend, P. and Davidson, N. (1980). *Inequalities in Health (The Black Report)*. Penguin, London.
25. Hayes, M.G. (1986). *Health Inequalities in Liverpool*. Liverpool City Planning Department, Liverpool.
26. World Health Organization (1981). *Continuing Education for Primary Health Care*. Report on a Seminar, San Remo. WHO, Copenhagen.
27. World Health Organization (1982). *The Place of Epidemiology in Local Health Work*. Offset publication No. 70. WHO, Geneva.
28. Horder, J. (1983). Alma Ata declaration. *British Medical Journal* **286**, 191–4.
29. Tudor Hart, J. (1981). A new kind of doctor. *Journal of the Royal Society of Medicine* **74**, 871–83.
30. McGuinness, B.W. (1980). Why not a practice annual report? *Journal of the Royal College of General Practitioners* **30**, 744.
31. Morris, J.N. (1975). *Uses of Epidemiology*. Churchill Livingstone, Edinburgh.
32. Ashton, J.R. (1984). *Health in Mersey – A Review*. Liverpool University Department of Community Health, Liverpool.
33. NACNE (1983). *Proposals for Nutritional Guidelines for Health Education in Britain*. The Health Education Council, London.
34. Coronary Prevention Group (1984). *Coronary Heart Disease Prevention, Plans for Action*. Pitman, London.
35. Committee on Medical Aspects of Food (1984). *Diet and Cardiovascular Disease*. Policy Report of the Panel on Diet in Relation to Cardiovascular Disease. HMSO, London.
36. Brackpool, J., Ramharry, S. and Ashton, J. (1984). *Shopping and Coronary Prevention in Liverpool – A Pilot Study*. Liverpool University Department of Community Health, Liverpool.
37. Brown, J. (1986). Causes of Death in Three Liverpool Wards. Student dissertation, Department of Community Health, Liverpool University, Liverpool.

38. Ashton, J. (1987). Making the healthy choices the easy choices. *Nutrition and Food Science* July/August, 2–5.
39. Ramharry, S., Constantinou, A. and Evans, J. (eds) (1985). *Regional Food and Drug Policy*. Mersey Regional Health Promotion Unit, Liverpool.
40. Carrall, T. (1987). *Exercise Policy Guidelines*. Mersey Regional Health Authority and the North West Sports Council, Liverpool.
41. Ashton, J. (ed.) (1984). *The Tranquilliser Problem in the Mersey Region*. Mersey Regional Health Promotion Unit, Liverpool.
42. Eldon St. Community Association (1986). The Eldonian Village. Eldonian Community Association, 31 Eldon Street, Liverpool L3.
43. Freeman, H., Dawson, G. and Parker, J. (1986). Mental Health and Housing Environs: A Psychiatric Planning and Design View. Paper given at Symposium on Unhealthy Housing, University of Warwick, Warwick.
44. Goodman, M. (1986). Health Implications of a Modern Housing Estate. Paper given at Symposium on Unhealthy Housing, University of Warwick, Warwick.
45. Smith, R. (1987). *Unemployment and Health*. Oxford University Press, Oxford.
46. Unemployment and Health Study Group (1986). Unemployment: A Challenge to Public Health. Occasional Paper no. 10. Centre for Professional Development, Department of Community Medicine, University of Manchester, Manchester.
47. Wescott, G., Swensson, P.G. and Zollner, H.E.K. (eds) (1985). *Health Policy Implications of Unemployment*. WHO, Copenhagen.
48. Langenback, R.R. (1986). Continuity and sense of place: the importance of the symbolic image. In *Mental Health and Environment* (ed. H. Freeman). Churchill Livingstone, Edinburgh.
49. Cochrane, A.L. (1972). *Effectiveness and Efficiency*. The Nuffield Provincial Hospitals Trust, London.
50. Welsh Heart Health Survey (1985). 'Pulse of Wales' Preliminary Report of the Welsh Heart Health Survey. Heartbeat Wales, Cardiff.
51. Ashton, J. (1988). Health promotion research and the concept of community. In *Research in Health Behaviour* (eds Anderson, R., Davies, J., Kickbusch, I. and McQueen, D.) Oxford University Press, Oxford.
52. Erikson, E.H. (1967). *Childhood and Society*. Pelican, London.
53. Slater, P. (ed.) (1976). *The Measurement of Intrapersonal Space by Grid Techniques*. John Wiley, New York.
54. Beol, N. (ed.) (1985). *Repertory Grid Techniques and Personal Construction*. Croom Helm, London.

7 The Health of Young People

According to the World Health Organization study group on Young People and Health For All by the Year 2000, adolescence is the period of transition from childhood to adulthood and is characterized on the one hand by efforts to achieve goals which are related to the expectations of mainstream culture and, on the other, by spurts of physical, mental, emotional and social development.[1] This transition, which in general covers the period from age 10 to 24, is characterized by the onset of puberty leading to full sexual and reproductive maturity, psychological development from the cognitive and emotional patterns of childhood to those of adulthood, and emergence from socio-economic dependence to relative independence.

Estimates suggest that 1445 million people are currently aged between 10 and 24 – one-third of the world's population. However, whereas in the developing countries the population of young people is increasing rapidly, in developed countries that proportion is decreasing and, as a consequence, the proportion of all young people living in developing countries is predicted to increase from 78 to 84 per cent by the year 2000.

In the United Kingdom, in common with many other developed countries, declining birth rates have led to much smaller birth cohorts, and, as a consequence, the proportion of the population aged under 16 years has declined from 25 to 20 per cent in 10 years.

Many people will presumably welcome the trend. This demographic change is likely to affect the whole style of popular culture and social policy preoccupation. Teenagers in developed countries have become famed for their clothes, records, noise and non-conformity, for flaunting their sexuality and energy and generally upsetting people who want a quiet life (Fig. 7.1).[2] One mass effect of the 25 per cent reduction in the number of teenagers, together with their reduced economic significance, is that youth culture is moving out of focus in favour of those with disposable income – the 'yuppie' generation in their early 40s and the segment of the retired population which has had the benefit of good occupational pensions.

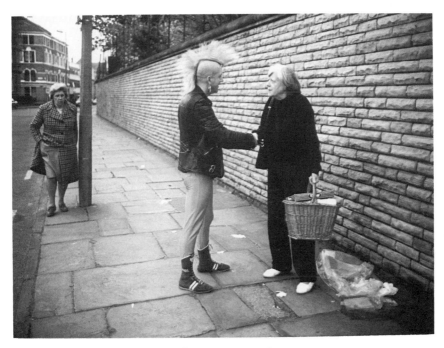

Fig. 7.1. 'Health for All' (photo © Chris Schwarz).

Quite major changes in some of the statistics pertaining to teenagers can be predicted, all other things remaining equal, e.g. fewer street crimes (mainly 14–17 year olds), fewer motor cycle accidents (about 1000 fatalities annually, predominantly 16–19 year olds), and fewer induced abortions (half of all abortions are performed on 16–24 year olds). But, on the other hand, there will be less energy around for all of us.

However unpopular young people often seem to be to the adult community, they are of fundamental importance to it. Adolescence is a form of biological, social and psychological revolution and renaissance which affects each generation and provides society with one of its main sources of creativity. It should be of no surprise that older generations have always complained about teenagers. As embryonic adults seeing the world with fresh eyes unencumbered by experience and compromise, adolescents are inevitably challenging and, through being so, can be a source of new ideas for solving the problems of the day. The friction which seems so often to exist with adults may say more about the complacency of adults than the impatience of youth.

In more traditional and perhaps more stable societies than those which now exist in most parts of Europe, the process of transition from an adolescent to a full adult member of the community, is often quite formalized through what can be seen as 'rites of passage'. The characteristics of such rites include the necessity for the adolescent to carry out and achieve a task which is difficult and challenging, and that on completing it he or she is accorded full adult status within the community; an enhanced and equal status which enables a person to play a full part.[3,4]

Such acceptance carries with it significant implications for the self-esteem and empowerment of each individual, aspects of affect and function which are increasingly seen by psychologists and health educators as central to the adoption of healthy life-styles. It is likely that the failure of the generation in administrative control to provide a supportive context for young people, and the general insistence on the part of adults on seeing young people as a set of problems, becomes a self-fulfilling prophecy.

Even before the very high teenage unemployment rates of the present time were reached, the opportunities for optimal transition to adult life were restricted in many countries to those who were able to enter a profession, skilled trade or family business. Many of the traditional forms of craft apprenticeship which fulfilled this role have gone, and even completing higher education is no longer a guarantee of being able to achieve adult status by obtaining work and financial independence.

In recent years the number of unemployed youths under 25 in the 24 nations of the European Organization for Economic Cooperation and Development (OECD) has reached more than 7 million.[1] In the largest countries in this group, young people accounted for around 40 per cent of the unemployed. Many young Europeans have never known what it is to hold down a real job.[5]

Against this background, the occasional headlines drawing attention to youth violence and a variety of socio-health problems should come as no surprise. What is perhaps surprising is the comparative lack of alienation of young people towards adult society rather than its existence. Certainly, the tendency of young people to associate in self-defined interest groups with identifiable clothing and life-styles, which may include various types of deviant behaviour, can be seen as attempts to give meaning and structure to their lives.

Assessing the Health of Young People

> Youth is a period of life when people are undergoing an intensive process of biological, sexual, social, educational and occupational development and maturing . . . Though mortality and morbidity are altogether low, this period of life is a time of high potential load for young people and is connected with some health risks and problems.[6]

Such a statement could be taken as lending weight to the feeling that the health of young people should not be a particular priority compared, for example, to that of infants and children or the elderly. There is, however, another way of looking at this, which leads to the conclusion that young people should be seen as possibly the most important priority.

The consequences of a blighted generation of young people will last for at least 60 years. These will be manifested directly in the effects of unhealthy life-styles, both now and in the future, through excess mortality, morbidity and burden of care in mid-life and old age. They will be manifested indirectly as a result of their inadequate parenting of their own children and lack of involvement in the care of the elderly and others to whom they might feel bound as part of the mutual social contract. The essence of this contract has been poignantly described by Titmuss in relation to the gift of blood donation, a gift characterized by absolute altruism.[7] Deprived generations grow up selfish and holding-on, rather than showing the sharing and caring which appears to be a phenomenon based on intergenerational trust and security.

The actual mortality rates for young people are low compared with those for infants and the elderly.[1] In historical terms and until AIDS became a threat to young adults, there had been dramatic declines in mortality in this age group and especially from infectious disease. In most developed countries, accidents, suicides and other external causes now constitute the major causes of death in adolescence. While the proportion varies from country to country, overall these causes are responsible for about one-half of all deaths.[1] However, in an increasing number of countries AIDS has now become the leading cause of death in young adult males.[8]

Pregnancy at an early age presents a particular danger for women and their offspring. This continues to be a threat to physical health in developing countries, but is comparatively unimportant in developed countries because birth control is available to teenagers; however, there is still a threat to mental and social well-being.

In general terms, the health risks to young people are those related to the consequences of any inexperienced person exploring new worlds, in this case the physical, interpersonal and intrapsychic environments. Inevitably, there will be casualties, but these casualties can be reduced if risk-taking is accepted as part of the process of adolescence, if adolescents are helped to equip themselves with the knowledge and skills necessary to optimize their control over their own situation, and if this is done in a supportive family and social context.

Despite an apparent awareness that youth health really needs to be considered in the round, there is a strong tendency to reduce it to its epidemiologically defined elements. Thus

relevant documents of the United Nations Organisation, the World Health Organisation Headquarters and the World Health Organisation Regional Office call special attention to the following problems of the health condition and health behaviour of youth:

- Accidents and behaviour risky to health
- Alcohol abuse and alcohol dependence
- Drug abuse and drug dependence
- Mental disorders, suicide and attempted suicide
- Disabilities and handicaps

- Sexual and reproductive health problems, uncontrolled pregnancy
- Acute respiratory diseases and other infectious diseases
- Caries
- Malnutrition

At the same time, it is pointed out that behaviours detrimental to health, especially widespread cigarette smoking, cause a predisposition to cardiovascular diseases and cancer.[6]

This approach, although it encompasses a number of the life-style areas of the World Health Organization European Targets, seems to lead to a narrow focus on vertical programmes of intervention. Such programmes tend to focus on one problem at a time and imply preconceived ideas of desirable outcomes, enshrining the values of health educators or those currently in political control. Where a horizontal or integrated approach is adopted the focus is commonly on applying that integrated programme within a single sector where young people are to be found, e.g. schools, health care or a youth service. The challenge of Health For All, of escaping from the didactic into the participative and from the single sector into real multisectoral approaches, seems to be rare.

Teenage Pregnancy as an Example of a Vertical Problem Struggling to go Horizontal

Over the past 100–150 years there have been changes in the physical and social aspects of adolescence.[1] The age of onset of sexual maturation has been decreasing, growth and physical development are proceeding at an accelerated pace and, until recently, there has been a trend towards greater ultimate adult size; however, in most countries there continue to be marked social class differences in the height and weight of school leavers.[10] The age of menarche in Europe has become earlier by 2–3 months per decade and there is a similar trend in the USA. Better nutrition and improved social and economic conditions are important underlying factors supporting this process.

In parallel with these changes in physical maturation have been changes in the social culture and life-style of young people, especially in developed countries. In the 1950s and 1960s the 'teenager' was discovered as part of the post-war 'bulge' generation. Labour was in short supply, teenagers enjoyed full employment and became a ready focus for commercial exploitation.[11] Their economic independence led to social and sexual independence, something which was assisted by the development of effective contraception in the form of the pill. Bury has categorized six specific reasons related to the trends in teenage sexual behaviour:

1. Changes in attitudes.
2. Changes in parental behaviour.

3. Rising incidence of marital dissolution.
4. Lessening influence of religion.
5. Influence of the media and of advertising.
6. Peer group pressure.

It also seems that the source of young people's information about sex is important and that the more open and informative parents are about sex, the less likely teenagers are to experience early intercourse.[12] It is against this background that birth control and related services for young people should be considered.

Most people now accept planned parenthood as an important and attainable goal. There is a considerable body of evidence that the birth of unplanned and unintended children is associated with major disadvantages for those children; disadvantages which have social, psychological and medical dimensions.[13–15] Teenage pregnancy is associated with a variety of physical problems for the mother and with increased perinatal and maternal mortality. From the economic point of view, as measured by the costs to society of unplanned pregnancies, family planning has been shown to be extremely cost-effective.[15]

The birth of an unintended child is much more common among teenagers than among older women and some of the underlying reasons for this involve the constellation of moral, psychological, educational, organizational and political factors surrounding community attitudes towards sexuality, health education and youth counselling services. In the United Kingdom, when a teenager marries, often as a result of pregnancy, the marriage has twice the prospect of breaking down compared with a marriage involving a woman aged 20–24 years of age.[17–19]

Although the increased availability of health education, contraception and abortion services during the 1970s and changes in the attitudes of the public at large and of health professionals have led to a decrease in the number of live births and unintended pregnancies at all ages, the position with regard to unmarried teenagers remains a cause for concern.[19] When teenagers become sexually active they are initially slow to use contraception and, therefore, continue to have an increased risk of unplanned and unwanted pregnancy.[21] However, teenagers are less likely to become pregnant and less likely to become mothers than they were in the early 1970s.[9,22,23]

During the 1970s the teenage pregnancy rate (15–19 year olds) in England and Wales fell from 63.1 pregnancies per 1000 in 1971 to 44.1 pregnancies per 1000 in 1981.[9,14] However, an increasing proportion of these residual pregnancies now result in induced abortion and this is worrying for a number of reasons. Quite apart from the absolute moral opposition to abortion which is held for example by the Roman Catholic Church, there is reason for public health concern about the increased risks faced by teenagers undergoing abortion as a result of the delays which they experience prior to obtaining their operations.[24–26] These delays result in teenagers having later operations than older women. Such later operations probably carry an increased risk of emotional and physical damage, including impairment of future fertility.[27]

The decrease in teenage conception rates seems to have occurred during a period when, if anything, teenagers have become more, not less, sexually active. Farrell's study in the mid-1970s in England found that by the age of 19 years approximately one-half of single women and two-thirds of single men had had sexual intercourse, a pattern which with minor differences seems to apply to similar developed countries.[9,27] In parallel with the recurrent concern which is expressed about the incidence and consequences of teenage pregnancy, is a concern about the effects of teenage sexual behaviour on the incidence and effects of sexually transmitted diseases, which are most common in the late teens and early 20s, on the risk of cervical cancer in later life and on emotional and psychological development.[17,29] The appearance of AIDS has added to this concern.

A Community Approach to Positive Sexual Health, the Prevention of Unintended Teenage Pregnancy and Infection by Sexually Transmitted Disease – The Swedish Experience

There has undoubtedly been a large extension of health education in recent years. However, it is likely that such education is only able to make its full contribution to the reduction of teenage pregnancy and sexually transmitted disease when it is part of an integrated community-based programme and supported by public policies which set out to influence the entire health field in relation to sexual attitudes and the expression of human sexuality. To achieve this the programme must be congruent with the values and aspirations of the community. Such a programme which has addressed itself to the prevailing spiritual, public, parental and professional dimensions and to the provision of services, as well as education, has been developed and implemented by more than half the Swedish counties.

Sweden has experienced 15 years of systematic effort to respond to the needs of young people, not only for sex education and contraception, but also for caring support and positive acceptance during their first adult relationship.[30,34] As expressed by Carl Gustav Boethius:

> when teenagers are blamed for going steady, they become desperate. When they have the experience of being accepted – when they feel that parents and teachers look with sympathy and joy at them and their boyfriend or girlfriend then they have the spontaneous feeling 'we must take care of this. We must live up to the confidence they have in us. We would even like to discuss the situation with them and maybe even take advice from them.'[32]

Underlying such a view is an acceptance both of sexuality as a positive force in relationships and of the fact that our children are indeed 'only lent to us for a short time.'[33]

The model which has been developed in Sweden is based on the necessity of 'breaking down the conspiracy of silence between the generations' and is aimed at creating community-wide initiatives which move and spread 'like rings on the water'. The general approach is through intensive residential workshops for key opinion formers, decision makers, role models, teachers, other professionals and counsellors of young people. The agenda for these workshops includes factual information about human biology, personal relationships and the family, pornography, prostitution and venereal disease. The methods used include lectures, role play, discussions, group work, theatre and film. The intention is to provide a non-threatening learning and working environment where attitudes may be explored, ignorance remedied and common ground sought.

Of particular value has been a short history of four generations in a farming community on the Baltic island of Gotland written by the district nurse and midwife from her own experience.[34] This simple account of how family life has changed within recent memory strikes a chord with workshop participants who can recognize that not all in the good old days was necessarily good and not all in modern times is bad; it seems to facilitate the creative process in a remarkable way.

Workshops like these are held throughout a county and involve people at town and school level. As a consequence, several hundred people have, in effect, become resource persons for programme initiatives, such as group discussions in school or the visits of teenagers to community clinics to familiarize them with the services which are available, and provide the opportunity for seminars aimed at raising sensitivity to the need for contraception to be considered as a joint responsibility within a relationship. This mainstream work is reinforced by events such as festivals and mobile services; the work is carried out with the active collaboration of the media from the beginning. In the Gothenburg programme, after 2 years of work a 1-week film festival was held in which a constantly changing programme of films about love and sex, romance and pornography provided the stimulus for a city-wide debate about the nature of sexuality and the appropriate community response to it.

With the focus very much on relationships and on 'Living Together' rather than on the mechanics of sex and contraception, the Swedish initiatives can be judged to have met with considerable success. Not only has there been a 40 per cent reduction in Swedish teenage conception rates, but this has been accompanied by falls in sexually transmitted disease, and in claims that drug abuse and delinquency are in decline.[9,35] The attempt to reproduce the Swedish model in the United Kingdom has not been so fortunate.

The Liverpool Project – A True Story

The total population of Liverpool Health District was 519,000 in 1981. This population has a very heterogeneous complexion with strong historical links to

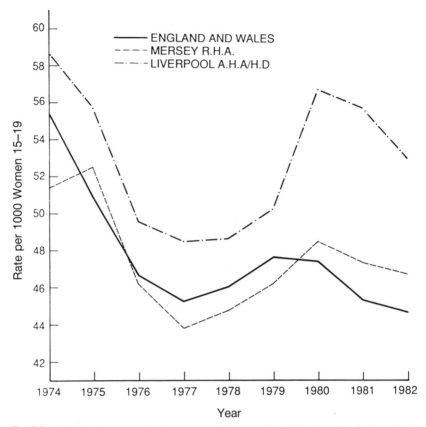

Fig. 7.2. Notifiable reproductive events (live- and still-births, plus induced abortions). Rates for England and Wales, Mersey and Liverpool, 1974–82.

Ireland and the influence of the Roman Catholic church is still strong within the city. However, the city has one of the highest teenage conception and illegitimacy rates and one of the highest teenage abortion rates in the country (Fig. 7.2).[36] Although there was an extensive network of Health Authority family planning clinics in Liverpool in the early 1980s, there was no special provision of family planning and youth advisory services for young people other than a limited service provided by a charity, the Brook Advisory Centre.[37] Provision for specialized clinics for young people was strongly recommended in a Department of Health memorandum on family planning services which proposed 'separate, less formal arrangements for young people. The staff should be experienced in dealing with young people and their problems.'[38,39]

A proposal for a community-based intervention to address the problem in Liverpool was commissioned by the Health Education Council in London in 1983. During the following 3 years a process was pursued which took account of the Swedish experience.[37,40] The attempts to develop a demonstration project, which would be acceptable both to the Health Education Council and to the relevant departments of central government, has to be seen against the continuing controversy generated by legislation on abortion and the focus on the prescribing of oral contraceptives to girls under the age of 16 years which arose as a result of the test case brought by Mrs Victoria Gillick to the House of Lords in 1984–5.[41] On the one hand, genuine concern over teenage pregnancy and sexually transmitted disease has led to a desire for action aimed at reducing their incidence, while on the other hand, there is anxiety by some that any efforts in this area will be construed as an encouragement to the undermining of notional traditional moral values.

In January 1981, Mrs Gillick had written to her local health authority requesting written assurance that in no circumstances whatsoever would any of her daughters (Beatrice, Hannah, Jessie or Sarah) be given contraceptive or abortion treatment while they were under 16 in any of the family planning clinics under their control, without her prior knowledge and irrefutable evidence of her consent.[42]

Having failed to obtain assurances which she required, Mrs Gillick began legal proceedings against her local health authority. In July 1983 she lost her case in the High Court and began to contest the ruling in the Court of Appeal. In December 1984 her appeal was upheld in the following terms:

> That the notice [of guidance] issued by the Department [of Health] . . . is contrary to law. That no doctor or other professional person employed by the first defendants . . . may give any contraceptive and/or abortion advice to any child of the plaintiff below the age of 16 without the prior knowledge and/or consent of the said child's parent or guardian save in cases of emergency, or with the leave of the court.*[1]

There followed a period of almost 12 months of extreme uncertainty. Youth advisory clinics reported a dramatic reduction in the numbers of younger teenagers seeking contraceptive advice, and family planning nurses reported that they had been prohibited from teaching in schools. An acrimonious debate was waged throughout the media with the new political right proclaiming the death of the permissive society and family planning workers and health educators struggling to mobilize middle of the road opinion to defend long fought for freedoms. This fight took place over the heads of the teenagers affected: the moralists against the professionals and the politically committed.

---

* 'In 1972 there were 1,490 births and 2,804 induced abortions among resident girls under 16; these figures are vivid reminders of the need for contraceptive services to be available for and accessible to young people at risk of pregnancy, irrespective of age. It is for the doctor to decide whether to provide contraceptive advice and treatment and the Department is advised that if he does so for a girl under the age of 16 he is not acting unlawfully provided he acts in good faith in protecting the girl against the potentially harmful effects of intercourse.'

The real losers in all of this must have been those teenagers who were newly becoming sexually active and who temporarily at least had lost access to those services which were controlled by the adults. Finally, the Law Lords ruled by 2 to 1 against Mrs Gillick, supporting the Department of Health appeal against the Appeal Court ruling of December 1984.

In initiating a process of consultation in Liverpool to establish a model programme against this backcloth, an understanding of the potential pitfalls was central to the consultation strategy adopted. It was felt to be essential from the start to establish a relationship based on trust between key community representatives, decision makers and professionals, which would provide a basis for people with widely varying beliefs to cooperate for the common good.

Underlying this resolve was an implication from London that Liverpool was a bad choice for such a project because Liverpudlians were thought in some way to be irrational and incapable of cooperating in a community project of this kind involving, inevitably, people of different persuasions working together. This was further complicated by the existence in Liverpool of a large Roman Catholic population. Naturally, this image was resented in Liverpool, and it was pointed out that the churches in Liverpool had made pioneering advances in ecumenicism in recent years.[43,44]

The most important initial work included the development of a structured process of consultation to establish prevailing attitudes among community representatives, decision makers and professionals towards teenage pregnancy and sexually transmitted disease, to establish whether there was support for a project and, if so, what the constraints and facilitating factors would be. A wide network of contacts and people committed to some kind of intervention was identified, including:

1. Young people, self-help and women's groups, and groups with special needs such as homosexuals.
2. Representatives of ethnic minorities.
3. Religious bodies (the Church of England, the Roman Catholic Church and the Jewish Synagogue).
4. Specific services for young people (counselling and guidance clinics, both statutory and voluntary).
5. Youth and community workers.
6. Social services for young people including specialist services, child care, fostering and intermediate treatment.
7. Education (teachers, advisers, school inspectors, parent support and teacher trainers).
8. Medical and nursing personnel, including those from obstetrics, genitourinary medicine, paediatrics, community medicine, general practice and family planning.

In all, about 50 people became involved and provided the basis for a 3-day residential workshop conducted along lines developed by the Swedish Board of Health, with the assistance of the British Family Planning Association

Education Unit and resource people from Sweden and China. The workshop consisted of small- and large-group sessions with the following objectives:

1. To make explicit the values of the participants.
2. To match up these values against participants' perceptions of the needs of young people.
3. To identify whether or not there would be general support for a demonstration project and to clarify the possible nature of such a project.
4. To identify those factors which might facilitate or hinder the success of such a project.

Detailed analysis of the feedback from workshop participants identified three essential sub-programmes of a demonstration project:

1. Education and training for interpersonal relationships, probably based on the Swedish model.
2. Socio-health services for young people.
3. Information and media resources.

In addition, the research which would be needed in support of a project was explored. Subsequently, specific recommendations for the sub-programmes were developed taking account of the special position taken in relation to the proposed project by the Roman Catholic Archdiocese. An important outcome of the workshop had been a statement by the representative of the Catholic Church which identified areas of common concern and agreement. This included, in particular, the willingness of the Archdiocese to cooperate in working to enhance and deepen personal relationships among teenagers and a statement supporting a programme of sex education in Liverpool schools. There was agreement about the desire to work against the exploitation of sexuality in the media and in advertising, to reduce the number of induced abortions among teenagers and to eradicate sexually transmitted disease. Differences between people on these issues concerned means rather than ends and the Archdiocese's delegates stressed the importance of considering the Roman Catholic response in the context of the beliefs and teachings of the Catholic community.

The importance of not seeing teenage sexuality in isolation from the overall condition of young people or of viewing young people as a problem to be tackled in an instrumental fashion was implicit throughout much of the workshop discussions. When it comes to teenage sex it seems that we are caught in a web of our own making. Many family planners appear to be motivated primarily by paternalistic, hygienist considerations rather than by the quest for real freedom, with its implication that people are trusted to make informed choices for themselves. The dilemma of healthism is well put by the savage in his conversation with Mustapha Mond in Huxley's *Brave New World*:

I want poetry, I want danger, I want freedom, I want goodness, I want sin.

'In fact', said Mustapha Mond (from the new world), 'you're claiming the right to be unhappy.'

'Not to mention the right to grow old and ugly and impotent; the right to have syphilis and cancer; the right to have little to eat; the right to be lousy; the right to live in constant apprehension of what may happen tomorrow; the right to catch typhoid; the right to be tortured by unspeakable pains of every kind!'

There was a long silence.

'I claim them all', said the savage at last.

Mustapha Mond shrugged his shoulders. 'You're welcome to them', he said.[45]

The medicalization of birth control which has followed the advent of oral contraception has reinforced the hygienist tendency. Also, we now have the bizarre situation where the promotion of condoms to prevent AIDS is acceptable but not to prevent conception, because AIDS has generally fitted in well with historic concepts of public health involvement in infectious disease control.

For adults as a whole, it is frequently difficult to steer a path between benign neglect and authoritarianism. This is particularly true for those of us whose cultures still have strong feudal overtones such as England, for those with an over-romantic view of life, as often seems to be the case in North America and wherever more primitive religious notions surface; a phenomenon which seems to be particularly common throughout the world at times of economic hardship.

The need to move from external to internal psychological directedness and control clearly carries with it a common fear of freedom. That when freedom is first tasted it can lead to license only reinforces the beliefs of those who are attached to their own bondage and would prefer others to remain likewise, as it makes them feel more secure.

Mrs Gillick's apparent distrust of her daughters can be seen as a projection of her own difficulty in trusting herself with freedom. The motives of a whole generation of Western leaders in consigning the current youth generation to the scrapheap may be similar but more complex. Economic discipline is one of the most primitive and potent forces there is. Mrs Thatcher and her Ministers have made frequent attacks on the 1960s generation, attacks which have often seemed to stem from resentment by a generation whose adolescence was marred by their growing up in the 1930s, before the teenager became the centre of attention.[11] In removing the economic importance of teenagers in the 1980s in favour of an older age group, there is in prospect another cohort of bitter adults reaping economic and social havoc in 20–30 years time. The systematic way in which a comprehensive national anti-youth policy has been developed in Britain since 1979 has been well described by Davies.[46] This policy extends from education, youth provision, training for work, employment opportunities and income maintenance, to justice and law and order.

In January 1986 the proposal for a demonstration project in Liverpool was rejected by the Health Education Council despite 3 years work, the expenditure of a considerable amount of money and the goodwill of a community of half a million people. Later, in 1986, the AIDS scare led to a dramatic about turn by the government in its attitude to public information and education about sex and sexuality, resulting within a short time in programmes and advertisements on television encouraging condom use, based on an acceptance of a harm-reduction rather than a prohibition strategy.

The Need for a Multisectoral Approach

In New York City community workers involved in the community gardens movement take any and every opportunity to create recreational areas and allotment gardens from pieces of vacant or derelict land.[47] These initiatives provide a focus for neighbourhood involvement and cohesion, drawing in people from the surrounding streets as volunteers. In one such instance, the workers became aware of the very high pregnancy rates among young teenagers helping with the garden and, as a result, began their own youth counselling service.[48]

In the old industrial cities of parts of Western Europe,[41] derelict land is abundant, jobs are scarce and teenagers become pregnant, apparently sometimes motivated by the transient attraction of the oldest legitimate role for a woman – pregnancy and motherhood. In reality, prestige and self-esteem are short-lived for a 16-year-old school leaver with no qualifications, skills or stable boyfriend. This situation underlines the importance of bringing derelict land back into use to provide the work and motivation which enhance personal expectations, and the possibility of young people taking control of their own lives; this is likely to include the choice to defer pregnancy until it can become part of a total satisfying life.

Writing in the *New York Times* in May 1985, Franklin Thomas, President of the Ford Foundation, made what appears to be a growing call for a national youth service.[49]

> Proponents of such a program share the conviction that young people represent a vastly underused resource that should be encouraged to offer itself in the service of our society, economy and national defense. They believe a system of youth service might help dampen the incidence among youth of drug and alcohol abuse, crime and vandalism, unwanted pregnancies and other symptoms of alienation. Most important, national service could be more than a repair shop for social damage or a means of keeping youngsters occupied: it could help them sort out their identities, build lifetime principles and develop a greater respect for self and society.

He went on to indicate a number of such programmes, usually with an ecological interest from around the United States. Ignoring Franklin Thomas' desire to associate such programmes with National Defence and the implication that society is always deserving of the respect of young people, this field of personal development related to intersectoral job-creation initiatives appears to be one which has so far been largely underdeveloped in Western Europe. Apparently, sound examples of such programmes can be found in both Canada and the United States.

Possible Models of Youth Programmes from North America[50]

CANADA WORLD YOUTH (CWA)[51]

Canada World Youth was founded in 1971 and arranges exchanges between Canada and third world countries. Although in some ways similar to the American Peace Corps and the British Voluntary Service Overseas, CWA differs in that it is actually an exchange programme. Perhaps this reflects the contrast between colonizer and colony. Between 1971 and 1984 the programme had involved 1000 Canadian communities and an equal number of communities overseas in more than 34 countries. In all, more than 7000 young people aged between 17 and 21 years have benefited from the exchanges.

Canada World Youth's objective is to allow young people and community members to share an educational experience through which they increase their awareness and acquire knowledge related to local and international development. Based on the knowledge acquired through the Canada World Youth Programme, the long-term objective is to encourage the young people and community members to participate more actively in local and international development with respectful concern for the environment and in a spirit of understanding between peoples.

Each exchange programme is between 6 and 8 months in length, half of the period being spent in Canada and the other half in the exchange country. Each Canadian participant is paired with a 'counterpart' participant from the exchange country and seven pairs of participants together with a Canadian group leader and an exchange country group leader constitute a group. Each group works together on a community development project which is sponsored by a host community. During the course of the orientation and participation in the programme, the following elements usually figure prominently: language, communication skills, critical judgement, leadership skills, understanding other cultures, social awareness, career choices and development (including food, health, education, ecology, population, volunteer work, cooperative systems, technology and disarmament as they relate to Canada and the world). In this way health promotion is incidental to much of the activity of the programme.

KATIMAVIK[52]

Katimavik is a national volunteer programme for young Canadians between the ages of 17 and 21. It was designed in 1977 to promote education and personal development, community awareness and knowledge of the country. Participants come from every region of Canada and represent a cross-section of the Canadian population. They join the programme to take part in a 9-month experience that involves working in three Canadian communities, living with other young people and learning new skills. In some ways it seems to resemble the British Community Service Volunteers.

The four fundamental objectives of Katimavik are as follows:

1. To help young Canadians acquire and develop skills that will enable them to contribute to the improvement of the quality of life in Canada.
2. To provide useful work training, as well as personal and community service experience.
3. To give young Canadians the opportunity to increase their awareness of Canadians' social and cultural diversity and their knowledge of a second official language.
4. To help them develop an appreciation of the environment in which they live.

Katimavik is based on a partnership between sponsoring communities and the volunteers. A total of 2000 young people take part, and exchange projects have taken place between Canada and California and Canada and France in relation to environmental conservation.

One notable feature of the Katimavik programme is the detailed attention given to training packages with considerable emphasis being given to health and fitness, language and environmental issues. Funding is derived from local communities as sponsors together with government money.

Katimavik is interested in exchange programmes with job creation or personal development programmes in Europe. An attempt to arrange such an exchange with a job creation scheme in Liverpool with the 'Health buses' floundered because the government agency involved held that personal development was outside its terms of reference.

PEACE CORPS[53]

Peace Corps, now in its third decade, was initiated as a phenomenon of the 1960s by President Kennedy. The goals as originally set by the American Congress have remained intact: to help developing countries to meet their needs for skilled men and women and to help promote mutual understanding between the people of the United States and those of developing nations.

There are now more than 6000 volunteers at any one time on placements throughout the world. In common with the British Voluntary Service

Overseas Programme, these volunteers are now likely to have a much higher level of skill than was the case 20 years ago. They offer skills in a variety of programmes: maternal and child health, family nutrition, freshwater fisheries, agricultural extension, teacher training, maths and science education, vocational training, small business consultation, forestry conservation and energy. Applicants must be at least 18 years old, with no upper age limits.

Clearly, with the trend towards taking on older, more skilled volunteers, Peace Corps has become of decreasing relevance to young people while perhaps becoming more relevant to the needs of the countries receiving volunteers.

Funding is predominantly from Federal monies. There would appear to be little scope for collaboration between Peace Corps and similar European programmes.

VISTA (DOMESTIC PEACE CORPS)[54]

Vista – 'Volunteers in service to America' – seems to resemble the British Community Service Volunteers and the Canadian Katimavik, but with much less emphasis on volunteer training for personal development than is clearly the case with Katimavik. During the past 15 years, 70,000 men and women have been volunteers with this programme, which is predominantly Federally funded.

THE FRESH AIR FUND[55]

The Fresh Air Fund, an independent, non-profit agency, has provided free summer vacations to more than 1.6 million disadvantaged New York City children since 1877. Originally started by the Reverand Willard Parson and financed to a great extent by the assistance of the *New York Tribune* and latterly the *New York Times*, using their papers as vehicles for fund-raising, the Fund now consists of two main programmes:

1. Camps in upstate New York which provide 2500 New York children aged 5–16 years with a 2-week holiday each year on a 3000-acre reservation owned by the Fund.
2. The Friendly town programme, whereby 9000–10,000 children are placed with families for 2-week visits. Such visits are frequently the beginning of life-long friendships.[56]

In recent years, there has been a growing interest in incorporating health education into the range of activities offered to the children during their residential stay.

URBAN ADVENTURES[57]

Urban Adventures is a small, non-profit agency specializing in experiential education by adapting the Outward Bound model of learning to a wide range of experiences and populations. It concentrates on programmes for minority high-school students, drop-outs and youths at risk. The agency has close working relationships with the community garden and ecology movement. Their philosophy is to encourage students to develop the skills and attitudes necessary for them to be able to take control of their own lives and become 'independent, productive, responsible, caring human beings'.

Adventure activities include rock climbing and ropes courses, canoeing, weekend camping trips, and the 24-hour urban experiences in the 'Big Apple'. Since 1979, Urban Adventures has worked with inner-city youths from South Bronx, East Harlem, Manhattan and Brooklyn in programmes designed to facilitate self-confidence, group communication and cooperation, or life skills and individuality.

Included within the scope of work are training programmes for educators, one-day experiential learning outings for all age levels, leadership training programmes, consulting services, outward-bound orientation and an agriculturally-based learning programme. The Agency also runs as Environmental Education Centre which is an operational organic farm. Its resources include a working solar heating display, a crafts centre, kitchen and classroom and outdoor activities centre.

A SPECIFIC INITIATIVE − TORONTO 2010[58]

Partly associated with Toronto's declared mission statement 'to make Toronto the healthiest city in North America', an initiative was taken to enable forty 14–19 year olds to make their own video about Toronto in the year 2010. The Project had two goals:

1. To introduce participants to a wide range of issues pertaining to living in and operating the city of Toronto now, in order to help them develop their vision of Toronto in the year 2010.
2. To teach participants technical and production skills which will enable them to produce a video depicting their vision for the city in the year 2010.

This video was presented in the city of Toronto and to high-schools across the city to encourage other students to develop further alternatives for a better and healthier Toronto.

Those students involved had the opportunity to increase their awareness by working directly with resource people from every area, political candidates, local celebrities and people on the street. They were able to develop a thorough knowledge of technical, creative and production skills using professional video equipment under the supervision of accomplished video specialists, develop public speaking, script writing and interviewing skills and experience the personal challenges of working in a heterogeneous group of peers. The project was intended to provide a sense of social history harnessed to a view of the future and the encouragement of participation.

A BILL OF RIGHTS FOR YOUNG PEOPLE[59]

We, the people of New York State, believe in the right of every child to:

1. Affection, love, guidance and understanding from parents and teachers.
2. Adequate nutrition and medical care to aid mental, physical and social growth.
3. Free education to develop individual abilities and to become a useful member of society.
4. Special care of the handicapped.
5. Opportunity for recreation in a wholesome well-rounded environment.
6. An environment that reflects peace and mutual concern.
7. The opportunity for sound moral development.
8. Constructive discipline to help develop responsibility and character.
9. Good adult examples to follow.
10. A future commensurate with abilities and aspirations.
11. Enjoyment of all these rights, regardless of race, colour, sex, religion, national or social origin.

Synthesis

Too often young people are defined as a problem and the analysis never goes further than to subdivide the type of problem which is currently felt to be fashionable and to prescribe a supposed appropriate intervention. As with many contemporary health issues, the task of refocussing upstream towards horizontal, integrative, multisectoral, prophylactic approaches seems to be the task which society finds most difficult.

The time is right for a positive strategy for young people to enable healthy teenagers to become healthy adults through enhancement of self-confidence and self-respect and an involvement with the wider community. Programmes of specific health education should be incidental to that task and not be an aim in themselves. Such a strategy needs to involve the commitment of government to meaningful youth employment, education and recreation and involve the collaboration of central and local government and statutory and voluntary agencies in producing policies for youth.

References

1. World Health Organization (1986). *Young People's Health – A Challenge for Society.* WHO, Geneva.

2. Cohen, S. (1973). *Folk Devils and Moral Panics – The Creation of Mods and Rockers.* Paladin, London.
3. Mead, M. (1963). *Growing up in New Guinea.* Pelican, London.
4. Mead, M. (1928). *Coming of Age in Samoa.* Pelican, London.
5. *Time Magazine* (1985). 19 August, No. 33, pp. 14–19.
6. *Healthy Lifestyles of Young People; Participation, Development, Peace* (1985). Elaborated and edited on behalf of the Regional Office for Europe of the World Health Organization by the Institute for Health Education of the German Hygiene Museums in the GDR. WHO collaborating Centre for Health Education.
7. Titmuss, R.M. (1971). *The Gift Relationship.* Allen and Unwin, London.
8. *Journal of American Medical Association* (1986). The impact of acquired immunodeficiency syndrome on patterns of premature death in New York City. **255** (17), 2306–310.
9. Jones, E.F. *et al.* (1986). *Teenage Pregnancy in Industrialized Countries.* Yale University Press, New Haven.
10. Townsend, P. and Davidson, N. (1980). *Inequalities in Health – The Black Report.* Penguin, Harmondsworth.
11. Ashton, J. (1983). Children of the Welfare State. *New Society* **64**, 109–110.
12. Christopher, E. (1978). Sex Education. *British Journal of Family Planning* **4** (1), 15–17.
13. National Children's Bureau (1984). *Teenage Parents: A Review of Research.* NCB, London.
14. Bury, J. (1984). *Teenage Pregnancy in Britain.* Birth Control Trust, London.
15. Campbell, R., MacDonald Davies, I., MacFarlane, A. and Beral, V. (1984). Home births in England and Wales in 1979. Perinatal Mortality according to place of delivery. *British Medical Journal* **289**, 721–4.
16. Laing, W.A. (1982). *Family Planning – The Benefits and Costs.* Policy Studies Institute, London.
17. Health Education Council (1983). *Contraception Programme.* The Health Education Council, London.
18. Rimmer, L. (1981). *Families in Focus.* Study commission on the Family. Family Policies Study Centre, London.
19. Haskey, J. (1983). Marital status before marriage and age at marriage: their influence on the chances of divorce. *Population Trends* **32**, 4–14.
20. Francome, C. (1983). Unwanted pregnancies amongst teenagers. *J. Biosoc. Sci.* **15**, 139–43.
21. Ashton, J. (1980). Sex education and contraceptive practice amongst abortion patients. *J. Biosoc. Sci.* **12**, 201–10.
22. Ashton, J.R., Machin, D., Osmond, C., Balarajan, R., Adams, S.A. and Donnan, S.P.B. (1983). Trends in induced abortion in England and Wales. *Journal of Epidemiology and Community Health* **37** (2), 105–10.
23. Ashton, J.R. (1983). Trends in induced abortion in England and Wales. *British Medical Journal* **287**, 1001–2 (Editorial.)
24. Ashton, J.R., (1980). Patterns of discussion and decision making amongst abortion patients. *J. Biosoc. Sci.* **2**, 247–59.
25. Ashton, J.R. (1980). Components of delay amongst women obtaining terminations of pregnancy. *J. Biosoc. Sci.* **12**, 261–73.
26. Ashton, J.R. (1980). The experiences of women refused National Health Service abortion. *J. Biosoc. Sci.* **12**, 201–10.
27. Ashton, J.R. (1980). The psychosocial outcome of induced abortion. *British Journal of Obstetrics and Gynaecology* **87**, 1115–22.

28. Farrell, C. (1978). *My Mother Said*. Routledge and Kegan Paul, London.
29. Ashton, J.R. (1984). *Health in Mersey – A Review*. Liverpool University Department of Community Health, Liverpool.
30. The National Swedish Board of Education (1977). *Instruction Concerning Interpersonal Relations*. National Swedish Board of Education, Stockholm.
31. National Board of Health and Welfare, Committee on Health Education (1978). *Living Together* – A Family Planning Project on Gotland, Sweden, 1973–1976. National Board of Health and Welfare, Stockholm.
32. Boethius, C.G. (1986). Personal communication.
33. Ashton, E. (1970). Personal communication.
34. Larsson, B. (1975). *A Gotland Family* (ed. Hanna Olsson). National Swedish Board of Health and Welfare, Stockholm.
35. Hollander, G. (1985). Personal communication.
36. Grey, P. *et al*. (1986). Trends in Teenage Fertility in Liverpool, 1974–1983. Unpublished background paper for the Liverpool Project. Department of Community Health, Liverpool University, Liverpool.
37. Ashton, J.R. (1984). *The Liverpool Project*. Report of a Feasibility Study produced for the Health Education Council, London. Department of Community Health, University of Liverpool, Liverpool.
38. Department of Health and Social Services (1974). *Memorandum of Guidance on Family Planning Services*. Section 'g', '*The Young*'. DHSS, London.
39. Department of Health and Social Services (1980). HN (80) 46. Family Planning Service Memorandum of Guidance. DHSS, London.
40. Ashton, J.R. (1984). *The Liverpool Project – The Consultation Documents*. Submission to the Health Education Council. Liverpool University Department of Community Health, Liverpool.
41. Ashton, J.R. (1986). Teenage pregnancy – a warning from Britain. In *Uitvliegen . . . Maar er niet invliegen. Tieners en seksualiteit*. Van Loghum Slaterus, Netherlands.
42. Childrens Legal Centre Brief (1985). *Young People's Rights and the Gillick Case*. Childrens Legal Centre, London.
43. *Faith in the City* (1985). The Report of the Archbishop of Canterbury's Commission on Urban Priority Areas.
44. Sheppard, D. and Warlock, D. (1988). *Better Together – Christian Partnership in a Hurt City*. Hodder and Stoughton, London.
45. Huxley, A. (1977). *Brave New World*. Panther, London.
46. Davies, B. (1986). *Threatening Youth – Towards a National Youth Policy*. Open University Press, Milton Keynes.
47. Fox, T., Koeppel, I. and Kellan, S. (1985). *The Struggle for Space*. Neighbourhood Open Space Coalition, 72 Reade Street, New York.
48. Flanagan, J. (1985). Personal communication.
49. Franklin, T. (1985). National Service for Jobless Youth. *New York Times*, 6 June.
50. Robbins, C. (1986). *Health Promotion in North America – Implications for the UK*. Health Education Council, King Edwards Hospital Fund for London.
51. Hebert, J. (1976). *The World is Round*. McClelland and Stewart, Toronto.
52. Katimavik, 2270 Avenue Pierre Dupuy, Cité du Havre, Montreal, Canada.
53. Peace Corps, 806 Connecticut Avenue, NW Washington, D.C. 20520, USA.
54. Vista, 806 Connecticut Avenue, NW Washington, D.C. 20520, USA.
55. The Fresh Air Fund, 70 West 40th Street, New York, NY 10018, USA.
56. Fresh Air Fund's Bronx-Amish Link (1985). *The New York Times*, 9 June.
57. Urban Adventures, 126 East 31st Street, New York, NY 10016, USA.

58. Toronto 2010, 342 Queen Street West, Toronto, Canada M5U 2AZ.
59. Young People's Bill of Rights, New York State Division for Youth, 84 Holland Avenue, Albany, NY 12208, USA.

Drugs and AIDS: A Case Study

The History

The initiatives taken on AIDS prevention from the Mersey Regional Health Authority (MRHA) Health Promotion Team have a clear historical development. They stemmed from the World Health Education Conference in Dublin in 1985. At the conference, as is probably usual, there were one or two outstanding papers: at this conference it was the presentation by Margo and Duprie on AIDS prevention. Surprisingly, because perhaps of its radical implications and political sensitivity, the significance of this paper was not really recognized in the conference report and press literature. The impact of this presentation led us to seek out Dr Margo (Director of Health Promotion) in San Francisco later that year and to invite him to Liverpool to participate in an intensive week-long lecture tour. The aim of the lecture tour was to sensitize decision makers and potential activists across the community to the issue of AIDS and present a model for organizing prevention programmes – *Agenda Setting*. While Dr Margo was in Merseyside, extensive media coverage started the process of public *Consciousness Raising*. In 1986, AIDS had not really been taken seriously and was still seen as a gay, American phenomenon that would never arrive in the UK – the 'Ostrich Phenomenon'.

This tour illustrates a simple and powerful device which can be used to get a health promotion initiative going, *the visiting expert*. We define such an expert as someone who comes from afar, far enough away not to be dismissed by people's automatic judgements, set or prejudice, and brings their own slides!

The San Francisco Model

To us the approach taken in San Francisco to AIDS prevention was distinguished by a number of important features:

- political organization at the community level,

- involvement of the community,
- creating lead organizations,
- extensive market research of risk groups,
- involvement of risk groups in prevention programmes,
- partnership between the statutory and voluntary sectors,
- creative use of mass media and their involvement in the prevention programme.

By 1986 the impact of the AIDS epidemic in the USA had been very marked, both in terms of its effect on people and the amount of Federal resources that were beginning to be released. There were some 25,000 people suffering from AIDS, half of whom had already died, and possibly another 1.5 million already infected with the HIV. The number of cases reported was doubling every 7 months. The psychological impact of the disease on the communities most affected was dramatic. Money was flowing in previously unimagined amounts into prevention, treatment and care activities (although this was nothing compared with what was to come). In New York State alone, $4.5 million had been allocated to the 3-year-old State AIDS Institute by the State government. Voluntary fund raising was gathering steam – over $3 million was collected at Elizabeth Taylor's benefit night in Hollywood, and more than $500,000 at the Metropolitan Opera Gala.

At this time we heard the same opinions expressed on several occasions during our visit to a variety of agencies in the USA. The two phrases that particularly stick in the mind were: 'we've never had so much money' and 'we had forgotten about communicable disease!' The AIDS epidemic forced people to remember and revert to the traditional *public health response*. In the USA, and most notably in San Francisco, a model of care was developing that typified a modern derivative of the classic public health approach built on community support and active participation.

We were told that the approach developed in San Francisco was distinguished from that developing in other cities in the USA by a number of features which are best illustrated by comparing the San Francisco model with the much less well-integrated approach found in New York at that time. The first contrast between the two cities in dealing with the problem was the lower level of organization of the gay community in New York. In San Francisco, the community had built up considerable political muscle. The second was the more manageable size of the city – hundreds of thousands compared with millions. The third was the size of the gay community in San Francisco, one estimate suggesting a gay population of 150,000. Fourth was the high number of alienated, disorganized and marginalized intravenous drug users in New York. Our impression of the outcome of these differences was, in New York, of a rather disjointed approach that lacked a high degree of community involvement and relied to some extent on professional and restrictive approaches that were out of touch with the groups on whom they were targetted. One of the major lessons of the times was the importance of gaining contact with all people whose behaviour put them at special risk; closing meeting places such as bath-houses, restrictive policing of prostitutes and increasing the prejudice against drug abusers, all have the effect of driving these groups 'underground' into isolation and greater risk.

Action in New York was, of course, not all bad, although it must be admitted that they failed, and have continued to fail to deal with the issues of AIDS prevention with intravenous drug abusers. In New York the learning curve was very steep. One of the key features was increasing state and city funding of the Gay Men's Health Crisis (GMHC), a non-profit educational and social service organization which was first established in 1981. With the help of this funding, and voluntary and charitable support, the range of services developed by GMHC was impressive. These fall into three categories – clinical, educational and legal – and are based on similar concepts to those developed in a more coordinated way on the other side of the continent.

In San Francisco, an integrated approach to care had developed, centred around a ward in San Francisco General Hospital and vigorous voluntary agencies such as the Aids Foundation and the SHANTI Project, both of whom act as lead agencies for effective community care and hospice programmes. The care at the hospital was organized largely by nurse practitioners who also dealt with the 'worried well' through triage and screening programmes. The atmosphere deliberately created on the AIDS ward was cheerful and relaxed. There was strong support for the staff to help them cope with the emotional stress of dealing with terminally-ill patients. However, the aim, through the hospice programmes at the SHANTI Project, was to allow patients to die at home, looked after by friends – a 'buddy' system – and a community care programme of support and caring. Staff at the hospital, in the local authority health department and in the various voluntary agencies were also heavily involved in local and national educational programmes. Much of the work dealt with issues of secondary prevention, safe sex, personal health and life-style programmes, public lectures and work with the media to ensure that ignorance was not the cause of prejudice against the infected and risk groups, and the training of 'buddies' and people in the community involved in all aspects of the care of people with AIDS. Clearly, with an estimated two-thirds of San Francisco's gay population already infected by the time large-scale prevention programmes began, it was considered too late for primary prevention.

This was the starting point for the programme to be developed in Mersey. The situation was very different: the gay community in the Mersey Region was much smaller and well hidden, with little organization and political clout. There was also a large heroin using community, but one which was considered on the whole not to inject. But the main difference was that the virus had probably not really arrived. Primary prevention was the obvious priority.

AIDS Prevention in Mersey: The Beginning

Following the agenda-setting visit of Dr Margo a head of steam had developed among activists in the local gay group, the health authorities and local authorities. Despite this the opportunity for action was limited, because the public still did not recognize AIDS as a serious issue in the UK, and this feeling seemed to extend to the government and to health authorities and, consequently, very little money was available. Given this background, we decided initially to take two tacks. The first was to form an AIDS education committee, membership of this *ad hoc* committee being made up of individuals and organizations who had expressed an interest in becoming involved. One of the underlying aims of the committee was to maintain the energy and enthusiasm of the activists identified. The second tack was to try to raise the consciousness of the public to acknowledge and understand the risks and the potential for prevention.

THE AIDS ADVERTS

With very little in the way of resources available, our major priority to educate the public seemed difficult if not impossible. Dr Margo's lecture series had only been partially successful in agenda setting, it had sensitized decision makers to the issue and gathered around us a group of volunteers and activists. However, no one was going to support any extensive action without feeling that there was public or government support. The two are, of course, closely linked and in a sense everyone was waiting for the government to act. We were not prepared to wait, for we did not want our region to follow the example of San Francisco, where the resources flowed when it was too late for primary prevention and the real action was focussed on helping people to live with dying.

To raise public consciousness fast and in a powerful way you do not organize lectures or use professional networks, you use the media! The TV and its immense audience, its immediacy and its powerful imagery, was the medium of choice. We had for some time been interested in running a media advertising campaign on the local TV channels using public service (free) time. Unfortunately, we had failed, usually for two reasons: either we were refused time or the adverts we presented for approval were rejected as likely to cause offence. We tried again. A series of three commercials produced by the Norwegian Health Directorate came to our attention. They were ideal for our purpose and only really needed translating into English. They consisted of humorous cartoons, they showed the letters of the word AIDS indulging in unsafe sex followed by safe sex imagery. In one of them a condom descended onto the erect I of the word AIDS. These commercials fitted our requirements perfectly; they were symbolic and could, we thought, be shown without offence while children were watching, they had high impact, their advice was detailed and factually correct, they were morally non-judgemental and, finally, they were humorous – they diffused the freezing fear and panic that is attendant upon the AIDS message. We submitted them for approval. The same thing happened again! Both the BBC and the local commercial channel refused to show them. Reasons of public taste and their sensitivity were given. However, underlying this, we felt that the media were unwilling to take on the issue without a lead and protection from the government. Almost back to square one!

There were two beneficial outcomes from this foray into the media world. The first was a further development of our media network – Mersey was defined as a place to go for comment and for media stories about AIDS and its prevention. The second followed from the refusal of the Independent Television Companies Association (ITCA) to accept the commercials. Immediately after this we released the story to the media and this resulted in the broadcasting of the adverts in the region, nationally and internationally as a news story.

In the end we were overtaken by events. By the end of 1986 the government had decided to start a large-scale AIDS advertising campaign. We still regret the time that was lost but, on the other hand, the media campaign was just what was needed. Despite their high moral content, the lack of concrete advice and the appeal to fear and panic these adverts had their effect, they legitimized the issue. We were on our way!

THE MERSEY AIDS EDUCATION GROUP

Initially, the committee consisted of people who had expressed an interest in being involved in the prevention programme. It was a device for not losing too much impetus while we got organized. An AIDS committee had been set up by the Regional Health Authority which pre-dated the Mersey Aids Education Group (MAEG), but this was a solely medical committee. It was concerned with treatment, care, testing and the safety of blood products. Some members of this group were not especially sympathetic to the involvement of the community, particularly the gay community in its activities. There was a tendency to see AIDS prevention as a medical issue and were not keen on any public profile. The model seemed to be to try to protect the public by secrecy. This again mirrored the early days of the epidemic in the USA, where they had to learn again how to run a traditional public health prevention campaign.

The separation that developed between the medical and the prevention aspects of the response in Mersey has never been dealt with fully and, to this day, like New York, we have not achieved the level of integration found in San Francisco. This is unfortunate, but perhaps this integration only comes when we have a significant number of cases of AIDS. Linked to the membership and direction of this medical committee, was the tendency for virtually all of what little money was available to be used in developing treatment facilities and for hospital staff protection measures. This was at a time when the obvious and overriding priority was to keep the virus out of a part of the country which had a very low level of sero-positivity to HIV.

With the advent of greater public recognition of the issue the MAEG began to grow in importance. The committee which was set up to advise the MRHA Health Promotion Team defined the approach and values of the AIDS prevention campaign. It was, in fact, the values which were to lead the campaign – values such as participation, confidentiality and a non-judgemental approach. In fact, many of the activities of the committee more represented and promulgated the values than had any direct or measurable effect.

The group grew and very soon had gathered representatives from most of the relevant statutory and voluntary agencies in the region, some 80+ members. Despite the normal management stricture against large committees the MAEG has worked well and continues to be a lively and committed group. With its mixture of officers of widely differing seniority, of representatives and volunteers, the group shares many of the features of a *network* rather than a committee, and this is probably the secret of its success.

VALUE-LED HEALTH PROMOTION

The main aims of the MAEG were to dispel myth and rumour, treat AIDS as a sexually transmitted disease which could affect almost anyone, and establish the use of safer sex (and other preventive practices) by all at risk in our community. The approach was to be pragmatic, participative and take particular note of the views, needs and circumstances of people at particular risk. The types of action recommended were as follows:

1. *Local co-ordination.* Each local health authority was recommended to join with other agencies including the local gay community to produce and implement a policy reflecting good practice. This stricture has to a large extent been followed, but again learning to follow a traditional public health approach has been a difficult process in hierarchical health care organizations dominated by professions.
2. *Market research.* To ensure that the needs of the communities involved were taken into account, the mass education campaigns should take a rigorous approach to researching target populations, situation, understanding and response. Educational materials and interventions were, where possible, to be rigorously pre-tested *with the assistance of the members of the target group.*
3. *Media activity.* Public education would require a high level of media exposure. In order to gain a sensible, well-informed approach in the media, journalists should be involved in the development of the campaign and encouraged to decide for themselves to take a responsible approach.
4. *Educational events.* Provision should be made to support and encourage local educational events, forums, workshops and seminars, to introduce AIDS education appropriate to age, development and need.

5. *Anonymous testing*. It was suggested that consideration may have to be given to establishing (correctly as it has turned out) anonymous testing sites where individuals can have an HIV test, with appropriate counselling, which is entirely under their control and they cannot be identified afterwards. This recommendation was based on the experience in San Francisco, i.e. to encourage people to contact services without fear of identification and the many issues concerned in confidentiality.

6. *Intravenous drug users*. Special programmes were to be established to ensure that i.v. drug users do not share injecting equipment, and practice safe sex.

7. *Condoms*. A particular feature of the programme was to popularize the condom.

Some Action

Although we had now set up the initial structure we did recognize that there was a need for action. Committees/networks are very good for information exchange and getting values accepted, but for a *new* activity they are not so good at action. The MAEG, we always recognized, could be a short-lived device to maintain interest. The activity required a focal point. We needed to find a person to run and organize the campaign, and the Regional Health Authority accepted the need for such an appointment; however, a number of factors – the sensitivity of the appointment, organizational inertia, the difficulty of finding a suitable candidate, etc. – combined to cause delay. In the meantime, there was an obvious need to develop some initiatives.

The initiatives developed at this time followed the general guidance of the MAEG approach. They fell into three broad categories: consciousness raising, work with and support to risk groups, and strategy. They included:

1. *Popularizing the condom*. A great many media stories were generated about popularizing and eroticizing the condom. On the whole, these took the form of low-cost, media-attractive events. Examples included giving condoms out at gay and straight nightclubs, explicit information and free condoms in the university newspaper, proposed surveys by medical students of the provision of condom machines in men's and women's toilets in city pubs, and the accessibility of family planning services to men. One of the events that failed to get off the ground was designed to copy a Swedish initiative.

In Sweden, the health authorities recognized that summer holidays, when young people migrate (often for the first time by themselves) to the south of Europe, were likely to be associated with sexual experimentation and, therefore, high-risk behaviour. To counter this they arranged for a special passport wallet containing risk reduction information and free condoms to be given to everyone purchasing a student's European Rail Pass. We had not got the resources to copy this and rail passes are not such a popular means of travel to the flesh-pots of the south, so instead we tried to arrange with our nearest international airport to allow us to distribute condoms and AIDS information to youngsters queuing to fly off for their Mediterranean holidays. Unfortunately, we could not get permission from the airport authorities, and after a variety of delays we were told that our activities would pose a 'security risk' and could not go ahead. Despite this we managed to gain valuable media coverage.

2. *Telephone lines.* We provided financial support for the development of telephone lines and crisis advice provided by the Merseyside AIDS Support Group, a local voluntary group. This group also produced literature tailored to the needs of the gay community and set up, again with our support, training courses for volunteers in telephone counselling and other care activities. This model was followed around the region by the local health authorities as new voluntary groups were formed.

3. *Market Research.* To gain an idea of the state of and trends in public opinion we commissioned a market research company to undertake three detailed telephone surveys of samples of more than 600 people across the region. The results of these surveys were useful both in producing media coverage and guiding the development of the campaign. The results showed that people were very well and accurately informed but that their knowledge was having little impact on their sexual (safe sex) behaviour. We also demonstrated that the differences in knowledge between social classes were small and disappeared completely during the AIDS Week on the TV, radio and in the press. During this week, AIDS information was extensively integrated into prime-time viewing and programming. It is a model of how to get public health information over to the vast majority of the public and shows that almost everyone can learn and understand quite complicated messages if they are presented in the right way, time and medium. Once the media campaign was completed some class differences reappeared with a small inverse association between class and knowledge. This probably shows that people who regularly read the quality press and watch minority TV are going to be better informed. This is not because higher social groups learn or understand better but because our information media themselves are class discriminatory. Access to accurate information and informed opinion is restricted because the popular media usually aim to entertain not to inform. Because of the high level of accurate knowledge we decided to reorientate our efforts and concentrate more on services and facilities aimed at reducing risk behaviour than on public education aimed at increasing knowledge.

Two Directions

Our appointment of the first Regional AIDS Co-ordinator in the country once again drew in considerable press interest to the appointment and to the issue. He took up the appointment with considerable energy, devoting much of his time to media activities and to activities with the gay community. Before we advertised the post we had decided that in order to maintain a San Francisco-style campaign our coordinator should spend some time in that city learning about, and becoming enthused with, the approach. In the end, he spent time in both San Francisco and New York and attended some of their specialized training courses. Having someone experienced in the type of training developed by SHANTI among others led our AIDS activity in a new direction. We began to set up training for carers: courses for nurses on AIDS awareness, training for volunteers as home care volunteers or as 'buddies'. There was considerable demand from the community for these courses. This shows that faced with crisis we do have an altruistic community. Once trained, however, there was some disillusionment because we had many more carers than people needing care.

In retrospect, this could have been predicted. We had broken our own stricture. Our initial analysis had told us to copy the values of the San Francisco campaign but not the details of its action. In San Francisco, the action, the public health response to AIDS, had begun too late for primary prevention, the only real 'cure' for AIDS. They had, therefore, had to make the best of it and concentrate on coordinating and humanizing care and trying to reduce any further damage. In Mersey, the presence of the virus was low, yet we had begun to copy the care experience, not the prevention experience of our model. Two further factors may have supported this. In this country at that time, the impact of the virus had been far greater on the gay population than any other group. The mood in that community had in consequence turned towards care and reducing discrimination. The other factor was that people seem to be much more familiar with the concrete and immediately rewarding aspects of caring, rather than prevention. The analogy has to be with the way we run our health services where the vast bulk of resources goes towards care and treatment not towards prevention.

We had fallen into our own trap! To redress the balance our approach took two directions. Our AIDS co-ordinator was becoming more and more interested in putting into practise the lessons he had learned in San Francisco. In the end we decided, by mutual agreement, to continue to support his work, but as an independent consultant. Clearing the decks in this way meant that the important training work would continue in an energetic and unfettered way and find its own base. We could now concentrate more on prevention.

The direction that we now took was different from San Francisco, although it had its origins in Dr Margo's original agenda-setting visit and picked up on the lessons of the market research we had carried out. It was to concentrate on providing the facilities and encouragement for people to change their sexual and other risk behaviour.

At one of Dr Margo's sessions Allan Parry, the Regional Health Authority's Drug Training and Information Officer, heard about efforts to reduce the risk of HIV transmission in intravenous drug users. Margo talked about the illegal shooting galleries where injecting equipment is shared and their efforts to get pushers to distribute clean equipment and/or information about sterilizing syringes and needles. All this was set against a background of illegality, the 'War On Drugs' and the 'Just Say No Campaign' being waged by the Reagan

Administration. Allan Parry was stimulated to think that there must be a better and more systematic way.

We placed greater significance on this line of thought as it became clearer that drug users, and not homosexual and bisexual men, were going to be the important gateway for the virus to the wider community. By 1988 the British Government was advised by its own expert technical group, the Advisory Committee on Drug Misuse Working Group on AIDS and Drug Misuse, that:[1]

> the sharing of injecting equipment which has become contaminated with infected blood is a major route of transmission of the virus and in some European countries the majority of cases of AIDS (Italy and Spain) or HIV infection (Scotland) have occurred through the use of contaminated injecting equipment.
>
> In the UK, as in many other countries, injecting drug misuse has so far been the route of acquisition of HIV for the majority of infected women, most of whom are of child-bearing age (the vast majority in Scotland). And infected women are now giving birth to children in significant numbers . . . several have already died.
>
> Infected drug misusers can transmit HIV sexually as well as by sharing injecting equipment. Since the vast majority of drug misusers in the UK are thought to be heterosexual, sexual transmission will be an important route from them into the general heterosexual population. In one study in New York, where the virus is well established amongst injecting drug misusers, injecting drug misusers were thought to have been the source of the virus in 87% of cases in which heterosexual activity was believed to be the mode of transmission.

The War On Drugs

In developing a New Public Health Approach to the issue of drug misuse and AIDS prevention we were fortunate to have a radical participative approach to drug misuse. Under the leadership of Allan Parry, the founder of the Health Promotion Unit's Regional Drug Training and Information Centre, and Dr John Marks, the consultant psychiatrist at the Liverpool Drug Treatment Clinic, a pioneering approach had begun.

Against a national background of abstinence as the chosen theory of treatment they had started from first principles and redefined the aims and objectives of this service. At that time they took as their primary aim to get misusers off drugs. To do this they had developed therapeutic approaches which aimed at a fairly rapid detoxification, leading to abstinence. The use of opiates and other drugs in the treatment was usually confined to help people get through the process of withdrawal. Allan Parry and John Marks, from their different backgrounds of youth work and psychiatry, began to analyse the real impact of this policy on the community. Their view was that abstinence approaches were failing to deal with the social, community and health issues associated with illegal drug use. Detoxification approaches tend to attract a small minority of drug users and may only succeed with people who are personally motivated to stop. Because of this the treatment services are out of contact with the vast majority of injecting users. Drug users continue to use dirty, harmful street drugs, damage their health through dangerous practices and put themselves generally at risk. They may get involved in crime, theft, prostitution and drug pushing to pay for drugs. All this puts a tremendous burden on the family, community and on law enforcement and other agencies.

To overcome these problems, and with the active involvement of the police and other agencies, it was decided to offer a range of treatments including a maintenance-based approach at the clinic. Maintenance with clean drugs of a known dose, it was argued, would bring people in contact with the service, reduce the reliance on illicit drugs, and basically keep people alive and relatively healthy until they came to the decision to stop. This approach was successful in bringing people in contact with the service and seemed likely to have other desired effects. So successful was the clinic it began to clog up and its drug budget grew to a level that was causing concern to the local health authority.

The service in Liverpool was not without its detractors. However, despite this, the runes were cast and the idea of a *harm reduction* approach had been established.

Harm Reduction and AIDS Prevention

With the growing incidence of HIV among drug injectors, it was clear that they should bear the responsibility not only of protecting themselves from harm, but also of preventing the spread of a potentially fatal disease to the rest of the population. From the beginning the emphasis was on involvement of drug misusers themselves in the solution. The services which developed tried to free themselves from the automatic value judgements often found and to offer a user-friendly environment. The implicit educational theory adopted was that change is most likely gained if the issues of the group involved are addressed and contact with, and the participation of, the target group for the public health initiative are gained.

The harm reduction approach to drug misuse had already demonstrated its power to gain contact with large numbers of injectors. To build on this, Allan Parry took the courageous decision to start a user-friendly syringe exchange and harm minimization service. Towards the end of 1986 the service began in the Regional Drug Training and Information Centre. It was extensively advertised on the streets by drug users themselves and the number of clients rapidly grew to about 1000 by the spring of 1988 (a large minority of all injectors on Merseyside).

When the scheme first started the staff were surprised at the number and health status of the clients. Previous estimates of the number of injectors in the Region had to be revised. And the myth that most people on Merseyside smoke heroin and do not inject it had to be re-examined. A number of the clients presented themselves in a very poor state of health. Poor injecting practices and adulterated drugs had wreaked havoc. A major part of the service was to give people advice on drugs, teach them how to inject properly and direct them towards clinical and other care services. Another service developed at the centre was anonymous HIV testing, i.e. clients could give whatever name they liked, so long as it was possible to identify their records. It became more and more obvious that the users of the scheme were not being dealt with effectively by the National Health Service and were in need of a new type of primary care service.

It was an obvious and outstanding success and it was copied in all 10 health districts across the region. This was not without its problems, for although the idea of offering injecting equipment was copied the factors which led to success were not. In some places schemes lacked the user-friendly approach and failed to take account of the needs of the clients. This highlighted, for us, a problem of innovation, that is 'How to extend beyond models of good practice without control of the staff and circumstances?' There is no easy solution to this question – we are still searching. All we do know is that in this process of dissemination there were considerable forces arraigned and allied against us, the most notable of these being the professionals adhering to a rigid model of professionalism. Sometimes it seemed to us that the world was peopled with the researcher who wanted to research the problem before (s)he started (this in the face of a life-threatening disease that was spreading as they pontificated); the drug worker who wanted to counsel people for an hour before (s)he gave away a single syringe; and the practitioner who denied the existence of injecting in their community. And this is not to mention those who campaigned against a harm reduction approach and the people and services involved with it. This is not meant to be a universal condemnation of professionals, for there were many that gave support. What it does show is that professional groups with their control, privilege and status to maintain may be part of the problem rather than its solution.

One of the final lessons of our approach to drugs and AIDS prevention is the importance of facilities and environments which facilitate healthier choices. Our market research of the general population had shown that behaviour, not knowledge, was the problem. With the drug users we did not set up an educational campaign, but a network of facilities which were accessible and where they could gain the means to live a healthier life.

Prostitutes and Primary Care

The Syringe Exchange Scheme demonstrated that drug injectors and users of such schemes are not a unitary category. Among the clients there were some drugs users who were prostitutes and also some prostitutes who were coming to the service to avail themselves of the free condoms supplied there. We recognized that drug-injecting prostitutes were a special risk group for the spread of HIV, and the centre staff encouraged this section of their clients to take condoms out on the streets for their colleagues. Our AIDS Co-ordinator arranged a public meeting for the women to come and discuss and become involved in AIDS prevention. No one turned up! Later, as the relationship developed, we began to find out about some of the issues faced by these women. We found that the women had not come to the meeting for a number of reasons, the most notable of which were suspicion of social workers and a fear of having their children removed from them. They thought that the meeting was organized by social workers and would be 'packed with do-gooders'. Having failed with the meeting we decided to move in a different direction, to build up the relationship and our knowledge further and develop facilities.

The reason for pursuing this was our growing concern that, together with intravenous drug users, prostitutes could be an important risk group for the spread of HIV and were in need of protection and support. Many professionals concerned with HIV prevention in the Western world believe that prostitutes, along with drug injectors, provide the main 'gateway groups' by which HIV spreads into the general population.

Accumulated evidence from studies of groups of prostitutes from around the world is beginning to provide a general picture of their risk of HIV infection. The most alarming evidence comes from countries in Africa, where HIV is predominantly spread by heterosexual transmission. In Central African countries, the vast majority of prostitutes tested are antibody seropositive.[2] In North America, there is a more variable prevalence of HIV infection among prostitutes. One study of seven different areas of the USA found that the prevalence among 835 prostitutes varied from nil in Las Vegas to 57 per cent in New Jersey.[3]

In Europe, reported levels of HIV infection among prostitutes to date show wide variations. Studies conducted during 1985–6 found no seropositives among 400 prostitutes in Nuremberg, 101 in Denmark, 84 in Amsterdam and 56 in Paris, and only 6 per cent of 200 registered prostitutes in Greece were found to be seropositive.[7] However, 12 of 52 (23 per cent) prostitutes investigated in Amsterdam in 1983–4 were seropositive.[8]

The work that started in Liverpool on this issue had two general directions. We recognized the need to develop further the relationship with the prostitutes and take our activities out on to the streets. We also recognized the need to understand the organization and distribution of prostitution and understand the issues with which prostitutes were faced. The latter was of particular importance because we were interested in pursuing with this group the same model of prevention as we had with the drug users, i.e. to provide facilities which are accessible, user-friendly and offer services which satisfy the needs of the clients and also make healthier choices the easier choices. From the start of this work, which again was led by Allan Parry, we thought that a new style of primary health care centre for this underserved group might prove a part of the solution.

It was obvious that we needed an 'outreach worker' to work with the prostitutes and undertake some 'quick and dirty research'. The choice of a candidate for such difficult and sensitive work was not easy. We wanted someone who was committed, would spend long hours on the streets, was street-wise, could get on well with the prostitutes and was sufficiently able and organized to do research. After some false starts we made an ideal appointment. Lynn Mathews was in no formal sense an academic. However, she proved to have all the qualities needed to do the special research work and produce the necessary reports. This appointment has proved that you do not have to employ a professional researcher for this type of research. In fact, we think that there are very few qualified researchers that could possibly have taken on this role.

Lynn took to the streets and collected data on both the statistics of prostitution and the views, experiences and needs of these women. She also began to distribute condoms, although these were eventually provided from one of the women's flats. She also offered some educational services, met and supported the new girls starting their career and encouraged the drug users into our services.

What did she find?

The average age of the 34 prostitutes surveyed was 26 years, with a range of 16–39 years. A notable shared characteristic was that 65 per cent had been in care and 65 per cent had been in prison. The women claimed to provide services to between 1 and 30 clients (mushes) a day, with an average of about 8 a day. However, the mean number of condoms used per day was five, although some of this difference may be due to non-penetrative sex acts rather than unsafe sex. Although 70 per cent of the prostitutes claimed to always carry condoms, 36 per cent admitted to being prepared to have intercourse with a client without using a condom, usually at the insistence of the client. Furthermore, 18 of the 25 women who lived with a non-business sexual partner said they had unprotected sex with these partners; 14 (41 per cent) were using injectable drugs (opiates in 12 cases). Six of the opiate users injected drugs and three of these admitted to sharing needles.[9,10] In short, these figures show a community at considerable risk.

The women were also asked about their contact with services, and which services they would use if available. Nine (24 per cent) of the women had never had a check-up for STDs, for such reasons as lack of confidentiality, unfriendly treatment, fear of losing children into 'care', and the amount of time it took. For those who did have regular check-ups, 18 (56 per cent) used the 'special clinic' at the local teaching hospital, and complaints about these services mirrored the reasons given for not attending by those women who had no check-ups.

The service most likely to attract prostitutes was a free condom facility, which 88 per cent would visit, followed by breast cancer screening (80 per cent). Almost 75 per cent said they would also be attracted by STD and HIV testing facilities.

This data and the other more informal feedback we received led us to plan a user-friendly health centre for prostitutes and drug users. The Maryland Centre was to be located on the edge of the 'block', the major area of street prostitution in Liverpool. This user-friendly and accessible centre would offer a variety of primary care and preventive screening services. It would provide treatment services, antibiotics and other drugs, syringe exchange, free condoms, an STD clinic and other primary care and screening services. We were aiming at creating a popular and value-free centre for providing care, help and education to underserved groups.

The other issues arising which were of a more intersectoral nature included:

- The way in which policing practices can drive prostitutes to pick up clients very quickly, so as to get off the streets and avoid arrest. Taking less care in the choice of clients puts the women at greater risk of violence and of being forced to practise unsafe sex.
- The way that the courts are involved in the cycle of prostitution. They impose large fines which the women can only afford to pay through further acts of prostitution.
- The need for illegal drugs can force drug-using girls to practise unsafe sex to get money or drugs from clients.
- The high proportion of the women who have been in council care as children and who seem to be dumped from care into the real world to look after themselves.

All of these are wider issues, ones which require public debate and/or the involvement of a variety of agencies. There is an obvious need to look at the issues of the decriminalization of drug use and prostitution. This is a big societal issue, but a change in the current laws and public attitudes may be needed to stem the spread of HIV. At a more local level, discussions will have to take place with the police and courts to change policing and sentencing policy. Social Services Departments will need to be encouraged to look at the effect of their 'care' activities and should at least ensure that all children in care have a better than average level of sex and AIDS education and are supported for some time after they leave the authority's care.

References

1. Advisory Council on the Misuse of Drugs (1988). *AIDS and Drugs Misuse, Part 1*. London, HMSO.

2. Murtagh, P. (1987). AIDS in Africa. *The Guardian*, 3rd February 1987.
3. CDC (1987). Antibodies to human immunodeficiency virus in female prostitutes. *Morbidity and Mortality Weekly Report*, 36, 157–61.
4. Smith, G. & Smith, K. (1986). Lack of HIV infection and condom use in licensed prostitutes. *Lancet*, December 13th 1986, 1392.
5. Krosgaard, K. *et al.* (1986). Widespread use of condoms and low prevalence of sexually transmitted diseases in Danish non-drug using prostitutes. *British Medical Journal*, **293**, 1473–4.
6. Coutinho, R. & van der Helm, T. (1986). No indication of HTLV III/LAV in prostitutes in Amsterdam who do not use drugs. *Nederlands Tijdschrift voor Genees-kunde*, **130**, 508.
7. Papaevangelou, G. *et al.* (1985). LAV/HTLV III infection in female prostitutes. *Lancet*, November 2nd 1985, 1018.
8. Cramer, A. (1957). Measures to combat AIDS among intravenous drug users. *World Health Forum*, **8**, 489–93.
9. Mathews, L. (1987). *Female Prostitution on Merseyside*. Liverpool, MRDTIC (mimeo).
10. McDermott, P. *et al.* (1988). *Prostitutes, Drugs and HIV Infection*. Liverpool, MRDTIC (mimeo).

9   Healthy Cities

Many streams of consciousness and endeavour have flowed together to create the Healthy Cities Project, a project first promoted by the European office of the World Health Organization in 1985.[1] After the Alma Ata Declaration in 1977, initial progress in creating a new momentum for public health had been slow and, despite the adoption of the Health for All Strategy by member States in 1981, for many countries the initiative appeared to stop there. In retrospect, it now seems that for the first 20 or 30 years of the World Health Organization, it was a common view in the more developed countries that WHO existed as a vehicle for the developed world to offer philosophy and advice to the developing world and that there were few implications for policy and practice at home. However, the global fuel crisis of the mid-1970s, a growing awareness of the McKeown hypothesis and the Lalonde initiative coupled with disallusionment at the returns from heavy investment in technologically-based medical care, gradually began to reinforce the message of Alma Ata that a reappraisal was needed everywhere. This was helped by the publication of the Health for All Strategy in a more accessible form in 1983.[2]

Interest began to be expressed in the Health for All Strategy in an increasing number of health and local authorities. In Britain, the Mersey Regional Health Authority adopted a Health for All framework in 1984 and it was soon followed by Bloomsbury District Health Authority and a cascade of others. A network of local authorities with health committees was established which became increasingly interested in the philosophy and framework offered by Health for All. Sheffield, Oxford and Nottingham were particularly quick to see the potential and to carry out special studies, produce Health for All reports or initiate interventions aimed at promoting health. In the voluntary sector, a variety of self-help and community development projects, which often had their origins in the social movements of the 1960s, continued to develop and came to be seen as of increasing relevance.[3]

A number of national governments, notably in Scandinavia, introduced legislation intended to reinforce the shift towards primary care and commis-sioned reports focussing on Health for All. However, generally speaking, there was frustration at the relative unwillingness of the medical sector to move towards a more social and less medical model of health. General practitioners, family doctors and primary medical care physicians seemed to have particular difficulty in seeing health promotion as anything other than specific preventive medicine procedures, such as immunization, screening or family planning services, or targeted health education aimed at achieving life-style changes in individuals.

A breath of fresh air came from Canada where the Lalonde Report seemed to have stimulated a variety of creative responses. Toronto had retained the same structure for public health services which had existed in the United Kingdom prior to the 1974 local government and health service reorganiza-tions. The city, therefore, continued to have a strong local authority public health department accountable to the local population through elected coun-cillors, and in the early 1980s it declared a 'mission statement' to make Toronto the healthiest city in North America by the year 2000.

It was in Toronto in 1984 that the idea of a healthy cities project first surfaced. A conference entitled 'Beyond Health Care' was organized in the city to review progress in the 10 years since Lalonde.[4,5] That conference also had its origins in a growing awareness of the need for 'healthy public policies' as compared with the tendency towards victim-blaming life-style approaches to health promotion which had become commonplace in many countries.[6] One particular paper entitled 'The Healthy City' provided a specific focus for a new synthesis which might 'bring together an ecological and holistic approach to health together with the WHO Health for All Strategy'.[7] The European office of WHO recognized that one implication of taking an ecological view of health was that human settlements as habitats might provide the focus and context for health promotion, which would make sense in a very practical way, and that this was particularly the case at the city level.

The Healthy Cities Project

The original intention behind the Healthy Cities Project was that by bringing together a small number of European cities to collaborate in the development of urban health promotion initiatives, it would be possible to promote models of good practice which were seen as relevant by other municipal administra-tions and would be picked up and copied or developed.

The project itself was seen as needing to demonstrate good practice by making the connections within WHO between the different departments, and the initiative for the project actually came from the Department of Health Education working together with the Department of Environmental Health. The inauguration of the project involved WHO working with the Nordic School of Public Health in Gothenburg, the Department of Community

Health at Liverpool University and an interdisciplinary planning group from throughout Europe and with an input from North America.

By concentrating on concrete examples of health promotion based on a commitment to equity, to community participation and intersectoral action, the Healthy Cities Project was seen as making the point at which the Health for All Strategy was taken 'off the shelves and into the streets of European Cities'.

That the city might be the most suitable base upon which to begin to build a New Public Health movement was clearly not a new idea. In nineteenth-century Europe and North America the rapid growth of industrial towns created the conditions under which epidemic disease was rife and it was the cities that responded to the challenge.[8,9] During that era it was common for public health initiatives at the city level to be local government responsibilities. The development of large bureaucracies based on the administration of medical and social care services and the illogical placing of preventive medicine and health promotion responsibilities within agencies without control over sickness-producing environments came later in some countries.

Today, although sometimes under attack from centralizing tendencies, the city with its own political mandate and often highly developed sense of civic pride is again in a unique position to pioneer a New Public Health. A central implication of the McKeown analysis is that most health is gained and lost outside the medical sector, often in those sectors over which local government has at least some influence or control. At the very least, the city represents the local accountable administrative level which has access to a wide range of resources and networks and can act as a facilitator, mediator and advocate for improving its citizens health.

By the year 2000, 75 per cent of Europeans and a majority of the world's population will live in cities or large towns. For most of us the urban setting will play a major part in determining our health. Throughout the world cities are to be found at many different stages of development. In some parts new cities are still being established and old ones continue to grow or to be remodelled. In others, once great cities are in a state of crisis and apparent rapid decline. Despite prophecies that the cities are doomed they remain in the front line of innovation and change and, for many, of our dreams of an urban Utopia; millions of people around the world still flock into cities when they are young. The challenge is now to find ways of renewing the momentum towards a high quality of life and Health for All for all city dwellers.

The familiar trends of growth and decay in cities have occurred in parallel with changes in traditional social structures – the decline of the three-generation family living in one place, the changing status of women, marriage, work and retirement, and radical changes in our personal and social expectations. Cities as the contexts in which so many people live out their lives have come to reflect the growing tensions and conflicting aspirations between those individuals and groups which inhabit them.

The need for a broad social view of health in the urban setting is becoming clear. The nature of medical problems has changed – infectious diseases have largely given way to heart disease, stroke, cancer, accidents and suicides, as the manifestations of a life-cycle which is out of step with those conditions under which we as a species evolved.

Beginnings

The first formal activity of the Healthy Cities Project took place in Lisbon in April 1986 when participants from 21 cities met to explore ideas about the healthy city and ways in which the project might usefully develop.[1] Subsequently, further meetings focussed on urban strategies for health and the information needed to monitor changes in city health.[10] The initially modest intentions for a project of 4–6 cities had to be changed to accommodate the enormous interest in the project and, by 1988, 24 European project cities were involved together with as many as 100 other European cities in national networks and networks of cities in Canada, Australia and New Zealand. The project was well on its way to global dissemination, had ceased to be a project and had become part of an urban movement (Fig. 9.1).

The intention behind the original project had been that it would last 5 years, by which time practical models of health promotion at the city level would be commonplace in Europe. The role of WHO was seen as a catalyst in the process of setting a new agenda for health, raising public awareness of the New Public Health issues and establishing models of good practice, drawing particularly on the Canadian and Mersey experience of health promotion.[11] By providing technical support to a small number of collaborating cities and creating opportunities for these cities to share their experiences, it was planned to pilot approaches which would have widespread applicability. The project was backed up initially by supporting centres in Liverpool and Gothenburg, with the intention that eventually many supporting centres would be developed as cities involved their local academic institutions in research and teaching appropriate to healthy cities work. The founding centres were involved in the production of background materials and resources for the project, and in facilitating research and teaching in relation to the project.

Steps towards a Healthy City

Agreement as to the precise nature of a healthy city is not necessarily easy to achieve. Certainly a healthy city is more than one which has good health services. One method which can be used to encourage fresh ways of looking at health in the city is by the use of scenarios workshops, a method which can also be used to explore contrasting visions of a healthy city and work towards building a consensus.[12] One of the original background papers for the Healthy Cities Project was a futures scenario for Liverpool as a somewhat unlikely healthy city, being one of the most rapidly declining cities in Europe at that

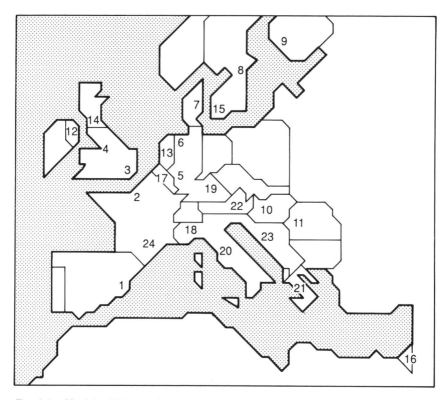

Fig. 9.1.   Healthy Cities Project.

1. Barcelona, Spain; 2. Rennes, France; 3. Bloomsbury/Camden, UK; 4. Liverpool, UK; 5. Dusseldorf, W. Germany; 6. Bremen, W. Germany; 7. Horsens, Denmark; 8. Stockholm, Sweden; 9. Turku, Finland; 10. Pecs, Hungary; 11. Sofia, Bulgaria; 12. Belfast, UK; 13. Eindhoven, Netherlands; 14. Glasgow, UK; 15. Gothenburg, Sweden; 16. Jerusalem, Israel; 17. Liege, Belgium; 18. Milan, Italy; 19. Munich, W. Germany; 20. Padua, Italy; 21. Patras, Greece; 22. Vienna, Austria; 23. Zagreb, Yugoslavia; 24. Montpellier, France.

time.[13] The thinking behind this approach is that although plans which take account of constraints are always necessary, to create a healthier future we must start with ideas and with a vision – those who start with 'realism' will never have vision.[14]

The idea of a healthy city incorporates the belief that the city as a place which shapes human possibility and experience has a crucial role to play in determining the health of those living in it. According to Hancock and Duhl,[15] two of the founders of the Healthy Cities Project:

a healthy city is one that is continually creating and improving those physical and social environments and expanding those community resources which enable people to support each other in performing all the functions of life and in developing themselves to their maximum potential.

This carries with it the implication that in a healthy city there is some kind of agreed 'common gameboard' and that, broadly speaking, people are pulling in the same direction; however, conflict and its creative resolution are also part of the healthy city. Yet each city is unique and has a life of its own, a soul, a spirit, even a personality; to understand a city it has to be experienced as a complete entity and as a place for living.[15]

At its most fundamental a city is unhealthy if it cannot provide its citizens with the basic necessities for life:

- safe and adequate food,
- a safe water supply,
- shelter,
- sanitation,
- freedom from poverty and fear.

However, these alone are insufficient and most people expect much more – a range of environmental prerequisites, economic, physical, social and cultural.

For most of recorded history cities have actually been very unhealthy places in which to live especially for their poorer citizens, and the implications in terms of inequalities in health and differential mortality rates are clear. It was in response to these problems that the Victorian public health movement came into existence and it is not by chance that town planning and public health have such a close pedigree.

It is perhaps not surprising that the awful conditions inspired thinkers to imagine urban Utopias as a stimulus to change, nor that visions of the future should have influenced the town planner Ebenezer Howard who developed the first 'garden city' suburbs in the United Kingdom at the end of the last century as a technical solution to the slums.[15]

In retrospect, many of the technical interventions of the recent past, such as housing estates and new towns, tower-blocks and fully-planned environments, are felt to have failed. Not only were people not consulted and involved in deciding their own destinies, but one of their most precious assets for health – their network of family and friends – was often negligently destroyed in the process. In creating a New Urban Public Health, the necessity to move away from paternalism towards partnership and citizen control is a central idea (Fig. 9.2).

The Healthy Cities Project contains five major elements:

1. The formulation of concepts leading to the adoption of city plans for health which are action-based and which use Health for All, health promotion principles and the 38 European targets as a framework.

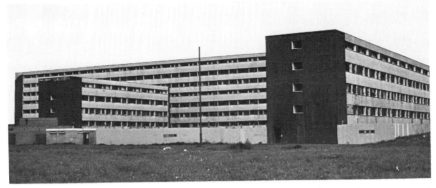

Fig. 9.2. One of the catastrophic housing developments built on the outskirts of Liverpool in the early 1970s. Tens of millions of pounds were spent on unacceptable high-rise flats that are now empty and awaiting demolition.

2. The development of models of good practice which represent a variety of different entry points to action depending on cities' own perceived priorities. These may range from major environmental action to programmes designed to support individual life-styles change, but illustrate the key principles of health promotion.
3. Monitoring and research into the effectiveness of models of good practice on health in cities.
4. Dissemination of ideas and experiences between collaborating cities and other interested cities.
5. Mutual support, collaboration and learning, and cultural exchange between the towns and cities of Europe.

In order to achieve these objectives, participating cities agreed to undertake seven specific tasks:

1. To establish a high-level, intersectoral group bringing together the executive decision makers from the main agencies and organizations within the city. The purpose of this group is to take a strategic overview of health in the city and unlock their organizations to work with each other at every level.

2. To establish an intersectoral officer or technical group as a shadow to the executive group to work on collaborative analysis and planning for health in the city.

3. To carry out a community diagnosis for the city down to the small-area level, with an emphasis on inequalities in health and the integration of data from a variety of sources including the assessment of public perceptions of their communities and their personal health.

4. The establishment of sound working links between the city and the local institutions of education both at a school and higher education level. Links at the school level can be explored as partnerships for learning, at the higher education level as partnerships for research and teaching. These latter links should not be confined to medical training establishments but should include any department or institution with an interest in urban health-related phenomena. Part of this work involves the identification of appropriate urban health indicators and targets based on the Barcelona criteria:[16]

- That they should stimulate change by the nature of their political visibility and punch through being sensitive to change in the short-term and being comparable between cities.
- That they should be simple to collect, use and understand, be either directly available now or available in a reasonable time at an acceptable cost.
- That they should be related to health promotion.

5. That all involved agencies should conduct a review of the health promotion potential of their activities and organizations, and develop the application of health impact statements as a way to make health promotion potential in different policy areas explicit. This includes the recognition that within a city there are many untapped resources for health, both human and material.

6. That cities will generate a great debate about health within their cities which involve the public in an open way and which works actively with the local media. This might include the generation of debate and dialogue using, for example, the interfaces which exist with the public, such as schools, community centres, museums, libraries and art galleries. A city's own public health history is itself often a powerful focus for debate and learning. Part of this work is the exploration of developing effective health advocacy at the city level.

7. The adoption of specific interventions aimed at improving health based on Health for All principles and the monitoring and evaluation of these interventions. The sharing of experience between cities and the development of multiple cultural links and exchanges underlies this work and is seen as promoting one fundamental goal of the World Health Organization, i.e. the promotion of world peace and understanding without which all health is threatened.

The emphasis of these tasks is on the provision of enabling mechanisms for health promotion to be developed through healthy public policy and increased public accountability; it is also on breaking down vertical structures and barriers and obtaining much better horizontal integration for working together.

Healthy Cities in Practice

Experience has so far suggested that firm political commitment to the healthy cities approach is essential for getting started. However, it is not uncommon to find a history of poor communication between the different sectors which need to work together either because of political differences or because of personality or professional conflicts. The Healthy Cities Project itself seems to provide a kind of neutral gameboard suitable for bringing together those agencies which should share a common interest in the health of the city. When the prime mover in introducing the Healthy Cities Project is not a politician but an officer or academic, the function of broker and of handing over ownership of the idea becomes particularly important. The process involved in this is one which is a key to all successful health promotion and community development work; it is strongly reminiscent of the style required of psychotherapists or counsellors and is well illustrated in the following Chinese poem:[17]

> Go to the people
> Live among them
> Start with what they know
> Build on what they have
> But of the best leaders
> when their task is accomplished
> Their work is done
> The people all remark
> We have done it ourselves

Tales and True Stories: The Beginnings of a Movement

Healthy city initiatives did not begin with the Healthy Cities Project. The community gardens movement in North America is a good example of the kind of ecologically orientated initiative arising from within communities which fits well into the philosophy of Health for All. Other examples include Rails to Trails in the United States and Sustrans in the United Kingdom, community organizations which are actively converting disused railway tracks to cycle and walking routes. In the South Bronx in New York, GLIE farms have ridden the wave of health foods and products by establishing a highly successful community business, growing and marketing fresh herbs to hotels and restaurants from a base in derelict industrial land within a community demoralized by unemployment, crime and drug abuse. Similar tales of urban regeneration are beginning to emerge from different parts of North America.[22] It is important to bear in mind the comparison between community-driven initiatives such as these and traditional initiatives of a paternalistic or centralist kind. What is needed for new initiatives like this is the active support and facilitation of the different agencies within a city.

A three-step approach to getting started has much to commend it:

Step 1: A presentation from someone with experience of the Healthy Cities Project in another city.*

Step 2: The initial presentation leads to the setting up of a small intersectoral working group to explore the feasibility of a healthy cities project and identify the problems; commonly the environmental health and city planning departments are involved at this stage.

Step 3: The establishment of a health policy sub-committee of the city council with a brief to take forward the Healthy Cities Project and to establish an intersectoral group and embark on the seven tasks.

Information and Measurement

The parameters by which one might measure the health of a city clearly span from the traditional ones of environmental protection and the quality of the physical environment through measures of mortality, morbidity and the quality of treatment and preventive medical services, into much softer though no less important measurements which define culture, participation, intersectoral collaboration and levels of mutual support. An outline list of suggested indicators was drawn up as a result of the first Healthy Cities Workshop in Lisbon in 1986:

1. Demography.
2. Quality of the physical environment including pollution, quality of the infrastructure and housing.
3. State of the local economy including unemployment levels.
4. Quality of the social environment, including levels of psychosocial stress and quality of social support services, strength and nature of local culture(s).
5. Personal safety.
6. Aesthetics of the environment and the quality of life.
7. Appropriate education.
8. Extent of community power and participation, structures of government.
9. New health promotion indicators, e.g. participation in physical exercise, dietary habits, alcohol and tobacco use.
10. Quality of health services.
11. Traditional health indicators (mortality and morbidity).
12. Equity.

The description of the health of a city along these lines requires a multidisciplinary approach and a recognition of the validity of subjective data. In addition to this basic list and to the Barcelona criteria, it has been argued that what is needed to stimulate action and change is a database adequate to allow an initial classification of cities on the basis of their major social and economic characteristics.[18] Unemployment rates, net population movements and travel

---

* 'A prophet is never recognised in their own country.'

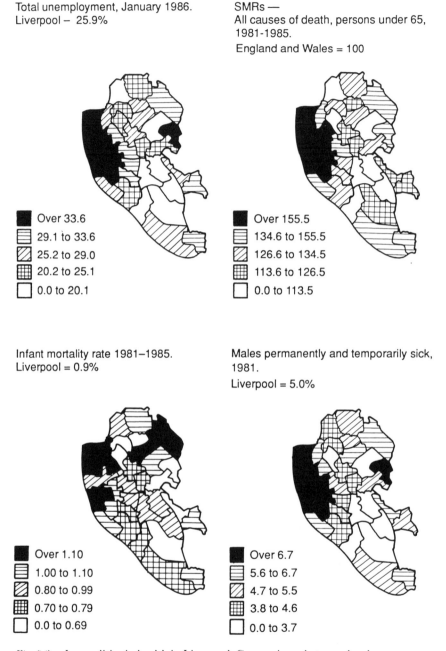

Total unemployment, January 1986.
Liverpool – 25.9%

SMRs —
All causes of death, persons under 65,
1981-1985.
England and Wales = 100

■ Over 33.6
▤ 29.1 to 33.6
▨ 25.2 to 29.0
▦ 20.2 to 25.1
☐ 0.0 to 20.1

■ Over 155.5
▤ 134.6 to 155.5
▨ 126.6 to 134.5
▦ 113.6 to 126.5
☐ 0.0 to 113.5

Infant mortality rate 1981–1985.
Liverpool = 0.9%

Males permanently and temporarily sick,
1981.
Liverpool = 5.0%

■ Over 1.10
▤ 1.00 to 1.10
▨ 0.80 to 0.99
▦ 0.70 to 0.79
☐ 0.0 to 0.69

■ Over 6.7
▤ 5.6 to 6.7
▨ 4.7 to 5.5
▦ 3.8 to 4.6
☐ 0.0 to 3.7

Fig. 9.3. Inequalities in health in Liverpool. Comparisons between local government wards for unemployment rates, standardized mortality ratios, infant mortality rates and permanent sickness rates.[21]

demand, as represented by hotel occupancy, coupled with available mortality, morbidity, biosocial and life-styles data related to inequalities in health between social groups should provide the starting point.

Even a preliminary analysis of quite traditional data may be sufficient to illustrate the extent to which inequalities in health are concentrated in small areas of urban conurbations (Fig. 9.3).[21]

Using computer analysis of the 1981 census and locally collected data, Liverpool City Planning Department has defined five standard data zones for the city which bring together spatially separate populations which share characteristics such as income level and housing tenure type.[19] However, it is clear that we need to further the third, social dimension of the WHO definition of health if we are serious about Health for All, and this will require development work.[20] The assessment of needs must also be parallelled by assessments of resources available, human and material, from both within and outside a community which could be liberated to promote health.

In the socially stressed Regents Park area of Toronto the local residents, together with the public health, housing and city estates departments, have combined to produce a community garden managed by a group of women from one of the tenements. This garden has provided a focus for community integration, active recreation, a nutrition education programme, not to mention the benefits which come from the production of fresh vegetables.

The potential for allotment gardens, small holdings and small-scale animal husbandry in urban areas is enormous, particularly in those towns and cities which have lost population and have an abundant supply of derelict land and unused buildings. The social, psychological, physical, nutritional, economic and environmental benefits of initiatives of this kind are obvious. What hinders them is frequently a lack of imagination or an over-rigid adherence to planning and public health rules and practices from another era. In Liverpool, as in all cities, there are many examples of such initiatives happening all the time; sadly it often seems they have had to be pursued either without the support of the public services or with their active opposition. One summer day in 1984 a derelict city-centre site in Liverpool became for many city children the seaside for the day with the assistance of a local contractor and his wagons bringing in sand. Happenings such as this are a magical and important part of the possibility of city life.[23]

The importance of creating cities fit for children is well illustrated by the Seattle KIDSPLACE initiative. Faced with the familiar pattern of population loss and increasing fears for safety, Seattle found itself in a position where an increasing number of people saw it as a city unsuitable to bring up children. The Mayor commissioned a survey in association with a local paper in which children were asked to identify how they felt about their city (Fig. 9.4).[21]

In addition, children completing the survey form were asked if they would like to be considered as a possible 'Mayor for the Day'. When the survey was analysed it was found to produce a very valuable perspective on the city and

A lot of people want to make Seattle a better place for kids. So I want to know what you think about different places in Seattle. What places do the words on this survey make you think of?

Fill out what you can. Have fun! Everyone who fills out and returns this survey will be entered in a drawing. The winner will get to be mayor for a day when school starts again. So let me know what you think of Seattle as a kids' place.

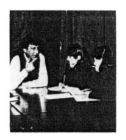

Mayor of Seattle

The name of my neighbourhood is

_____

What things or places do these words make you think of? Write your answers.

Example:

Wet GREENLAKE	Smells good	mysterious
Dirty	SAFE	QUIET
Beautiful	Sad	Friendly
FUN	Peaceful	Unfriendly
BORING	crowded	BUSY
UGLY	Smells bad	HELPFUL
DANGEROUS	noisy	TIRING

I think the best place to go in my neighbourhood is _____

I think the best place to go with my parents is _____

My favourite place in the city is _____

My parents' favourite place to go **with me** is _____

If I were Mayor, the first thing I would do to make Seattle a better place for kids is

_____

_____

generated ideas about how Seattle might act to make itself much more of a 'KIDSPLACE'. Subsequent to the selection of a children's Mayor, mechanisms have been developed for consulting with children to obtain their views on local policies which affect them. 'KIDSPLACE' has been picked up and copied in a number of the European Healthy City Project cities including some in Scandinavia, Germany, the Netherlands and Spain.

Initiatives in Project Cities

By 1988, the European Project cities had mostly reached the stage of setting up intersectoral groups and carrying out their community diagnoses. Some had already moved on to proposing specific initiatives. From Gothenburg came the story of a successful reduction in road accident mortality and morbidity by linking data from the hospital casualty departments with that from the police, and using it in the city planning and engineers departments to review the road system in a much more sensitive way than can be done by just relying on road death statistics.

From Horsens in Denmark came news of the establishment of a project shop, a citizen committee and a debate about Health for All. A proposal was put forward for an international children's workshop to bring together school classes from project cities, as a manifestation of international cooperation and understanding. Many cities began to produce reports on inequalities in health. Liverpool and Rennes collaborated in the first international exchange when teams of 13-year-old footballers, together with political and technical personnel, began the process of cultural exchange at the local citizen level which may grow and bloom. In Liverpool, specific proposals were developed for local healthy city initiatives, such as the designation of one of the most deprived and unhealthy areas of the city as a Healthy City Action Area with the intention of mobilizing on an intersectoral basis to reduce inequalities in health. Other initiatives include an integrated strategy for recreation and a campaign to reduce the number of accidents involving children. Major national healthy city conferences have been held in a number of countries, including the first United Kingdom Conference which was held in Liverpool in March 1988. True stories and tales have begun to emerge, and the exchange of ideas and experience is well under way (Fig. 9.5).

The Limits to City Action

There is a limit to what can be done at the local level, whether it is a city, town or neighbourhood. The policies which are needed to promote and protect public health are wide-ranging and at different levels of aggregation. To tackle the programme of work identified in the Liverpool Declaration at the first United Kingdom Healthy Cities Conference will require action at a national and international as well as at a local level (Appendix 2).

Fig. 9.4.   The Seattle KIDSPLACE survey questionnaire.

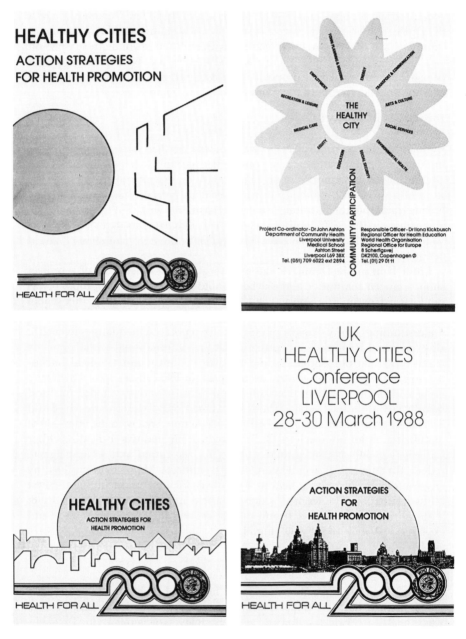

Fig. 9.5. From the general to the specific: as the Healthy Cities Project developed so the form of the city outlines became clearer. The flower as a project symbol represents intersectoral action founded on public participation.

The importance of the project has been to assert the need to think globally and act locally in the first instance. A great deal can be achieved in that way. The power of a global network of towns and cities rests in the potential for generating national and international policy from the bottom up through collaboration and the use of a large international network. The fruits of that collaboration should begin to be evident by the year 2000.

References

1. Ashton, J., Grey, P. and Barnard, K. (1986). Healthy Cities – WHO's New Public Health initiative. *Health Promotion* **1** (3), 319–23.
2. O'Neill, P. (1983). *Health Crisis 2000*. WHO, Copenhagen.
3. Smith, C. (1982). *Community Based Health Initiatives. A Handbook for Voluntary Groups*. National Council of Voluntary Organisations, London.
4. *Beyond Health Care* (1985). Proceedings of a working conference on healthy public policy. *Can. J. Public Health* **76** (suppl.), 1–104.
5. Lalonde, M. (1974). *A New Perspective on the Health of Canadians*. Government of Canada, Ottawa.
6. Hancock, T. (1986). Lalonde and beyond: looking back at "A New Perspective on the Health of Canadians". *Health Promotion* **1** (1), 93–100.
7. Duhl, L.J. (1986). The healthy city: Its function and its future. *Health Promotion* **1**, 55–60.
8. World Health Organization (1986). *Healthy Cities – Action Strategies for Health Promotion*, First Project Brochure. WHO, Copenhagen.
9. Chave, S. (1987). Recalling the Medical officer of Health (eds M. Warren and H. Francis). King Edward's Hospital Fund, London.
10. World Health Organization (1987). Background papers to Healthy Cities meetings in Goteborg and Barcelona, WHO, Copenhagen.
11. Ashton, J., Seymour, H., Ingledew, D., Ireland, R., Hopley, E., Parry, M., Ryan, M. and Holbourn, A., (1986). Promoting the New Public Health in one region. *Health Education Journal* **45**, (3), 174–9.
12. Hancock, T. (1988). Healthy Toronto – A Vision of a healthy city. In *Healthy Cities – Concepts and Visisons*. A resource for the WHO Healthy Cities Project Department of Community Health, Liverpool University, Liverpool.
13. Ashton, J.R. (1988). *Esmedune 2000. A Healthy Liverpool (Vision or Dream)*. Department of Community Health, Liverpool University, Liverpool.
14. Barnard, K. (1986). Lisbon Healthy Cities Symposium Notes of Closing Address on Behalf of the Planning Group. WHO, Copenhagen.
15. Hancock, T. and Duhl, L.J. (1986). Healthy Cities: Promoting Health in the Urban Context. A background working paper for the Healthy Cities Symposium. Portugal, 1986. WHO, Copenhagen.
16. World Health Organization (1987). *The Healthy Cities Project: A Proposed Framework for City Reports*. Discussion paper for the WHO Healthy Cities Symposium, Dusseldorf, June 1987, WHO, Copenhagen.
17. Chabot, J.H.T. (1976). The Chinese System of health care. *Tropical Geographical Medicine* **28**, 87–134. Quoted by Keith Tones in WHO (1987), *Education for Health in Europe*. A report on WHO Consultation on co-ordinated infrastructure within a Health Promotion Strategy. WHO, Copenhagen.

18. Flynn, P. (1987). Health indicators: context and the next steps. A background paper for the Indicators meeting of the Healthy Cities Project, Barcelona, March 1987. WHO, Copenhagen/Liverpool City Planning Department, Liverpool.
19. Liverpool City Planning Department (1984). *Social Area Study. The Results in Brief.* City Planning Department, Liverpool.
20. Brown, V. (1985). Social health in a small city. Paper presented to the 12th World Conference on Health Education, Dublin, September 1985. Health promotion Branch, Australian Capital Territory Health Authority, PO Box 825, Canberra ACT2601.
21. Liverpool City Planning Department (1986). *Inequalities in Health in Liverpool.* City Planning Department, Liverpool.
22. Rodale, R. (1988). *Visions of Regeneration.* Paper given on the United Kingdom Healthy Cities Conference, Liverpool, March 1988.
23. Henri, A. (1974). *Environments and Happenings.* Thames and Hudson, London.
24. Mayor's Survey (1984). *KIDSPLACE – Technical Report.* Seattle, Washington.
25. Knight, C. and Ashton, J. (1988). Proceedings of the First United Kingdom Healthy Cities Conference, Liverpool, March 28–30, 1988. (in press).

Appendix 1 Proposed Summary Indicators and Targets for the 12 Mersey Health Promotion Priorities

Priority	Availability status	Proposed summary indicators			Target
		Available now	Analysis required	Development work required	
1. Planned parenthood (WHO targets 1–4, 7, 8, 13–17, 18)		15–19 conception rates; proportion of conceptions resulting in live- or still-birth by age	—	Context statement	1. That by the year 2000 the conception rate for 15–19 year olds in all districts should be 14/1000 or lower
2. Prevention of sexually transmitted diseases (WHO targets 1, 2, 4, 10 13–17, 18)		Gonorrhoea infection rates by age and sex	—	Context statement	2. That by the year 2000 the increasing trend in gonorrhoea infection rates should have been reversed
3. Antenatal care including genetic screening and counselling (WHO targets 1, 2, 4–8, 13–17, 18)		Perinatal mortality rates	Proportion of women attending for antenatal examination by 3 months since last menstrual period	Context statement	3. That by the year 2000 the proportion of infants of low birthweight in the most disadvantaged ward of the district should be the same as that of the most advantaged ward and the perinatal mortality rates should similarly be equalized

Proposed summary indicators

Priority	Availability status	Available now	Analysis required	Development work required	Target
4. Child health and immunization (WHO targets 1–5, 7, 13–17, 18)		Immunization coverage levels	Height and weight of adolescents at school leaving age	Context statement	4. That by the year 2000 there should be no indigenous measles, poliomyelitis or congenital rubella
5. Prevention of death and disability from accidents and environmental causes (WHO targets 1, 2, 4, 6, 11, 13–17, 18–25)		Number of days when NO_x and SO_2 exceed WHO guidelines Home ownership by tenure type Proportion of households suffering from overcrowding	Home accident mortality and hospitalization rates Road accident mortality rates and hospitalization rates Industrial accidents, mortality and hospitalization rates Recreational accident, mortality and hospitalization rates Number of episodes of chemical pollution of water supply per annum Area-based patterns of food contamination and air, noise and environmental pollution	Aesthetic acceptability of the taste of domestic water Proportion of the population who find their domestic and/or working environment excessively noisy on a regular basis Number of homeless people Proportion of people who are dissatisfied with their current housing for structural or social reasons	5. That by the year 2000, deaths from accidents of all kinds should have been reduced by at least 25 per cent through intensified effort to reduce traffic, home, occupational and recreational accidents 6. That by the year 1990 all districts should have fully staffed departments of environmental health in local authorities with adequate mechanisms for public consultation and liaison with health and other relevant agencies 7. That by 1990 a clear picture of chemical pollution risk to the domestic water supply should have been established and a plan

drawn up to eliminate it, that measures will have been developed to assess consumer satisfaction with the taste of drinking water and regular consumer surveys begun to be carried out. That by the year 1995 chemical pollution of the water supply should have ceased to occur and public satisfaction with the taste of drinking water should exceed 95 per cent of the adult population

8. That by the year 1990 there should be no days in the year on which NO_x or SO_2 levels exceed WHO guidelines

9. That by the year 1990 the increasing trend in episodes of food poisoning should have been reversed and a system of training courses on the nutrition aspects of food established nutritional for food producers and for food handlers in retail outlets and cafes in both the public and private sector

Availability Priority	status	Proposed summary indicators Available now	Analysis required	Development work required	Target
					10. That by the year 1995 the major health risks associated with the disposal of hazardous wastes should have been eliminated and bathing beaches within the region should all reach EEC standards
					11. That by the year 2000 the proportion of households suffering from overcrowding in the most disadvantaged ward should be the same as that in the most advantaged ward, measures of satisfaction levels with housing, recreation space and noise levels will have been developed and regular surveys commenced, and the upward trend in homelessness will have been reversed
					12. By the year 1995 all employers will have made adequate arrangements to

			monitor work-related health risks and have agreed a prevention strategy with their workforce and with surrounding populations
6. Dental health (WHO targets 1–4, 13–17, 18)	Decayed, missing or filled teeth profiles for 5- and 16-year-olds by sex	Context statement	13. That by the year 2000 the decayed, missing and filled teeth ratio at age 5 years in the most deprived ward of the district will be as good as that in the most advantaged
7. Specific aspects of life-style related to premature death (WHO targets 1–4, 6, 9–19)	Unemployment rates Proportion of children receiving free school meals Proportion of school leavers continuing into higher education Household car ownership level Premature years of life lost and hospital bed days used by cause	Consumption patterns of alcohol, tobacco, prescribed tranquillizers and of illegal drugs by age and sex Exercise participation rates by age and sex Local area nutrition based on NACNE recommendations Height and weight ratios on a local population profile basis Local morbidity	14. That by the year 2000 mortality from diseases of the circulatory system in people under 65 years of age should be reduced by at least 15 per cent and the death rates in the most disadvantaged ward should be the same as those in the most advantaged 15. That by the year 2000 the current rise in male suicide and attempted suicide rates should be reversed and the decline in female rates should be sustained

| | Proposed summary indicators | | | | |
Priority	Availability status	Available now	Analysis required	Development work required	Target
				patterns and use of primary medical care by reason Perception of street safety	16. By 1990 all districts should have systematic programmes of health education to enhance the knowledge motivation and skills of people to acquire and maintain health, and each school should have at least one teacher designated as having responsibility to coordinate health education. Within each district, either provided by the health authority, the local authorities or both, there should be an effective health promotion unit adequately resourced to provide full support for the Health for All Strategy including health advocacy 17. By 1995 in all districts there should be established trends in positive health behaviour such as balanced nutrition, non-smoking, appropriate physical activity and good stress

management. Indicators of these trends should be available at at least ward level. The differences between the most advantaged and disadvantaged wards in health knowledge and behaviour and biological status should be narrowing

18. By 1995 in all districts there should be established downward trends in health-damaging behaviour, such as over-use of alcohol and pharmaceuticals, use of illicit drugs and dangerous chemical substances, and dangerous driving and violent social behaviour. Indicators of these trends should be available at a ward level and differences between the advantaged and disadvantaged ward in health knowledge and behaviour and in biological status should be narrowing. By the year 2000 the proportion of the population living in the most disadvantaged ward

Priority	Availability status	Proposed summary indicators		Development work required	Target
		Available now	Analysis required		
					engaged in satisfying work should be the same as that of people living in the most advantaged ward
8. Effective contol of high blood pressure (WHO targets 1–4, 6, 9, 13–17, 18)		Mortality and admission rates from stroke by age and sex		Context statement	19. By the year 2000 death rates from stroke within each district will be reduced by at least 15 per cent among those aged under 75 years, and the death rates from stroke within the most disadvantaged ward will be the same as those in the most advantaged
9. Early detection of cancer (WHO targets 1, 2, 4, 6, 10)		(a) Mortality rate for carcinoma of cervix and breast (b) Mortality rates for carcinoma of testis (c) Mortality rates for carcinoma of bowel and for melanoma by sex	Staging at time of diagnosis of specified malignancies	Context statement	20. By the year 2000 mortality rates in each district from cancer of the cervix, breast, testis, bowel and skin should be reduced by at least 15 per cent and the mortality rates from each of these cancers in the most disadvantaged ward should be the same as those in the most advantaged ward

10. Reduction of disability in the elderly (WHO targets 1–4, 6, 9, 11, 12, 13–17, 18)	Permanent sickness levels	Assessments of everyday living Context statement	21. By the year 2000 permanent sickness levels in the most disadvantaged ward of the district should be as low as those in the most advantaged ward
11. Dignity and comfort at the time of death (WHO targets 1, 13, 14, 18)	The dying: pain relief, physical comfort, psychological well-being Relatives and friends: satisfaction with patient management, psychological coping Context statement		22. By the year 2000 all those dying who are in contact with health and social services should be able to choose where they spend their last days and wherever that is should be able to expect optimal pain relief, physical comfort and psychological support from professionals
12. A healthy mind in a healthy body, positive health (ALL WHO targets, but, especially 13–17 and 18–25)	Context statement Psychological and social measures of well-being and measures of supportive public policy as overall context statement		23. That by the year 2000 the ability of people living in the most disadvantaged wards of the district to lead a socially and economically productive life should be the same as those living in the most advantaged ward

Appendix 2.   The Liverpool Declaration, 30 March 1988

WORLD HEALTH ORGANISATION
HEALTHY CITIES PROJECT

THE LIVERPOOL
DECLARATION
ON THE RIGHT TO HEALTH

Equity in Health

Community Participation

Partnerships for Health

Health Promotion

Primary Health Care

Research for Health

International co-operation

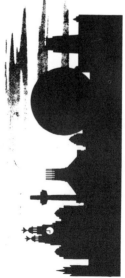

HEALTH FOR ALL

The Liverpool Declaration was produced by the Healthy Cities Inter-Sectoral
Committee, for ratification at the UK HEALTHY CITIES CONFERENCE held in
Liverpool on 28-30 March, 1988

THE LIVERPOOL DECLARATION

"At least I know this, that if a person is overworked in any degree they
cannot enjoy the sort of health I am speaking of; nor if they are continually
chained to one dull round of mechanical work, with no hope at the other
end of it; nor if they live in continual sordid anxiety for their livelihood; nor if
they are ill housed; nor if they are deprived of all enjoyment of the natural
beauty of the world; nor if they have no amusement to quicken the flow of
their spirits from time to time; all these things, which touch more or less
directly on their bodily condition, are born of the claim I make to live in
good health".

William Morris, 1884

BACKGROUND

The UK Healthy Cities Conference was planned by the agencies whose
collaboration forms the basis of Liverpool's involvement in the World
Health Organisations (WHO) Healthy Cities Project. Its purpose was to bring
together people from towns and cities in the UK to share ideas and
experiences in setting an agenda for the new public health in urban
situations. Two major aspects of this aim are the development of
collaborative healthy city plans and the promotion of a healthy cities
network of UK towns and cities committed to achieving health for all their
citizens. This Declaration represents a third aspect: Liverpool's agenda for
the new public health.

PRINCIPLES OF HEALTH FOR ALL

In seeking to achieve health for all citizens of the United Kingdom, we
acknowledge and confirm these fundamental principles, expressed in
the WHO "Global Strategy for Health for All by the Year 2000" (1981) and
the WHO European Region "Targets For Health For All" (1985).

THE RIGHT TO HEALTH
Health is a fundamental human right and a worldwide social goal.

EQUITY IN HEALTH
The existing gross inequality in the health status of people is of common
concern to all countries and must be drastically reduced.

COMMUNITY PARTICIPATION
People have the right and the duty to participate individually and
collectively in the planning and implementation of their health care.

INTERSECTORAL COLLABORATION
Governments have a responsibility for the health of their people which
can be fulfilled only by the provision of adequate health and other social
measures. The political commitment of the State as a whole, and not
merely the ministry of health, is essential to the attainment of health for all.

HEALTH PROMOTION
The starting point in changing lifestyles is to recognise that to a
considerable extent health depends on the political, social, cultural,
economic and physical environment. The first aim is therefore to provide
opportunities and develop capacities for adopting healthy lifestyles.

their area of residence, their physical abilities and their sexual orientation. In asserting people's rights to equity in health, we assert also their rights to fairness of treatment in all of these areas. These rights include their access to:

- adequate income, in or out of paid employment
- safe, warm, sound, affordable housing
- healthy, cheap, accessible food
- worthwhile, safe, properly rewarded work
- cheap, ecologically sound public and private transport
- freedom from sexual or racial harassment
- equal respect regardless of personal circumstances
- safe, planned, health enhancing environments
- leisure facilities and social support networks
- comprehensive, properly resourced public services

In actively promoting these rights we will work towards major reductions in the current inequalities in health.

COMMUNITY PARTICIPATION

We acknowledge the necessity for meaningful public participation in all processes and activities that affect people's health.

Health for all cannot be achieved without participation by all. A crucial element in becoming healthy is taking control over one's life. This has to involve empowering people by offering them a voice in the decisions that affect their health. Among other things, it implies opening up the membership of all bodies, at all levels, which take such decisions within the public sector; legislation may be necessary to achieve full participation. Decentralising management structures can be an important prelude to inviting participation. Policy decisions should also be informed by surveys of public attitudes and priorities. Empowering individuals to take part in activities affecting their health involves choosing policies and allocating resources that make the healthiest choices the easiest choices; once we have achieved this, any necessary educational processes are straightforward. In seeking participation, however, we also acknowledge the freedom of people to make choices and hold views on health with which we disagree.

INTERSECTORAL COLLABORATION — PARTNERSHIPS FOR HEALTH

We will work with all agencies and groups whose activities are relevant to the promotion of the public health.

Most of the major influences on health lie beyond the scope of health services. Despite this fact, there has been little real shared development

PRIMARY HEALTH CARE

Primary health care forms an integral part both of the country's health system, of which it is the central function and main focus, and of the overall social and economic development of the community.

INTERNATIONAL COOPERATION

Where health is concerned no country is self-sufficient; international solidarity is required to ensure the development and implementation of health strategies and to overcome obstacles.

In addition to describing the principles of Health For All, the WHO Global Strategy reminds us that 'in conformity with the recognition by the United Nations General Assembly of improved health should be channelled into sustaining economic and social development, and economic and social development should be harnessed to improve the health of people'.

TURNING PRINCIPLES INTO ACTIONS

THE RIGHT TO HEALTH

In recognising every citizen's right to good health, we accept the responsibility carried by all agencies, throughout our society, to take account of the public health costs of all their activities.

Practically all of the activities of agencies in our society can affect the public health. Such agencies include central and local government, health and education authorities, the non-statutory sector, employers, landlords, academic bodies: the churches, communicators: everyone taking part in the production and consumption of our goods and services, our values and attitudes. If health for all is to be achieved we must complement the economic audit which accounts for the financial costs of these activities with a social audit which assesses their health and other human costs. Without this social accounting for the health costs of public and private decisions, the right to health is an empty goal.

EQUITY IN HEALTH — THE REDUCTION OF INEQUALITY

We reject all forms of discrimination that reduce people's chances of good health, and accept the challenge of substantially reducing current health inequalities.

There are many aspects of peoples lives which contribute to the substantial and increasing health inequalities in the United Kingdom. These include, amongst others, their sex, their social class, their skin colour, between agencies at central or local levels of plans and strategies for promoting public health. We acknowledge the need for genuine joint planning for health for all; this must start from a consideration of the health needs of the people and 'work backwards' to the institutional means of meeting them. Such a joint approach to public health is required both between government departments and between local agencies and groups.

HEALTH PROMOTION

We acknowledge our collective responsibility to promote and create healthy physical and social environments, and to facilitate people's choices of healthy lives.

Health promotion is a constant theme in public policy, since both are concerned with improving the quality of peoples lives. We must be active in promoting awareness of this fact, and in working to make healthy the environments in which people live, work and enjoy leisure. People must also be given the resources and the information to make healthy choices. This involves a sensitive understanding of the responses of different social groups; traditional health promotion has often increased social inequalities in health.

PRIMARY HEALTH CARE

Primary health care must become the central function and main focus of our national health service.

Primary health care is the promotion of health and the provision of health care within communities. It is based on active partnerships between primary health care workers and the people, and on teamwork between primary health care workers and the most specialised elements of health care, and hence should be the main focus of health systems. In order to achieve these aspirations, embodied in the Declaration of Alma-Ata, we will strive towards:

- the direction of new resources toward primary health care
- the demystification of primary health care through patient participation groups, self-help groups, libraries, courses and other community resources in health centres
- the promotion of teamwork between all primary health care workers
- the provision of services sensitive to peoples needs such as well person clinics, nurse practitioners and community health workers
- localising the organisation and planning of primary health care to the neighbourhood level

INTERNATIONAL COOPERATION

As health promoters in a rich nation, we acknowledge our shared responsibility for the health of the world.

We wish to play a full role in Healthy Cities and other WHO networks which contribute to the health of all the world's peoples. In addition to material aid, we can fulfil this role:

- by actively opposing the export of unhealthy products
- by resisting the export by UK interests of practices harmful to the health of people in other countries, such as unsafe working conditions, inappropriate promotion of drugs or baby foods
- by protecting and providing for the health of migrant workers, refugees and victims of torture who come to the UK

RESEARCH

We will encourage in all relevant ways the research necessary to achieve health for all

We shall not achieve our goals without considerable developments in researching the public health. Much work is required if we are fully to understand the nature of the many inequalities in health. The development of social audit, accounting and investment poses a major challenge. Little is understood of the mechanisms of community participation in health. Joint approaches to public health planning and to healthy public policy require evaluation. If we are to move towards primary health care (and away from primary medical care), we must first demonstrate its greater effectiveness.

As well as new research agendas, health for all requires new styles of research, such as participatory methods which involve the affected communities in the design, implementation and action stages of research into their health; and research instruments which are sensitive to people's own health perspectives. Monitoring and surveillance of the public health will require new measures and indicators. All of the above will together constitute the development of a new social epidemiology which will refocus away from the diseases of groups of individuals and towards the health of populations. And of course, this development will not occur without the allocation of the necessary resources.

We seek the support of all people of the United Kingdom for this Declaration. We are sure that with that support, we can move confidently towards health for all.

Appendix 3   Black Declaration

Liverpool has one of the longest established black communities within Britain. Despite this, the economic, social and political position of black people within the city has not improved with time. Research by the area profile group Commission for Racial Equality and the Runnymede Trust, amongst others, clearly point to racism in the form of institutions preventing black people from gaining access to goods and services and taking their rightful place within society.

The healthy cities conference and the project, has to address itself to racism. In order to obtain health for all by the year 2000; the following has to be incorporated:

1. The development of policies, practices and procedures must ensure that black people have access to health care within Liverpool.
2. Equality of treatment.
3. Equality of employment opportunities.
4. To raise and maintain the level of awareness among workers within health on issues that face the black community.

On the issue of housing and future initiatives in this field, a concerted effort must be made to confront the endemic racism with this service provision:

1. Ethnic record keeping – in order to have accurate information base.
2. The setting of targets in order to combat inequality.
3. Training of staff on the issue of race.
4. Review of recruitment policies and procedures.
5. Employment of specialist staff.

On the issue of employment – the objective of any initiative must primarily evolve from a perspective of social and economic development within the Black community. There is therefore a need to:

1. Canvass and collate the skills of the black community.
2. Match these skills with the present employment market.
3. The setting up of positive action training schemes.
4. Action research.

The above points, when taken in conjunction with the recommendations for housing, can only be achieved with the targetting of financial resources, well thought out initiatives and the full participation of the black community within the decision making process.

All this needs to be set in an anti-racist context. It is only when these issues have begun to be addressed that HEALTH FOR ALL can become a reality.

Index

racism, 43
Rails to Trails, 160
Reagan, R., 45
re-orientating Health Services, 26, 32
rehabilitation, 22, 59
Rennes, 156, 165
representative democracy, 27, 43, 44
research, 30, 159
rest and recreation, 30, 33–6, 59, 66–7
review process, 60–1
Rhine pollution, 94
rickets, 65
risks to health, 22, 62
Robertson, J., 94
Royal Commission on the National
    Health Service, 31

San Francisco, 136–8
sanitation, 23
school health services, 17
shoe-leather epidemiology, 53
scientific medicine, 1
Scott-Williamson, G., 32
Seattle kidsplace, 163–5
security of employment, 52
self-care and self-help, 10, 23, 48
sex/gender, 12
sex/sexuality, 46, 118–27
sexually transmitted disease, 59, 72–3
SHANTI Project, 138
Sheffield, 152
shopping and health, 97–101
Sigerist, H., 92
single parents, 9
skills, 26, 100–1
skimmed milk, 65, 102–3
Skoal Bandits, 65
slave trade, 50
Slob of the Year, 65
smoking, see tobacco
Snow, J., 53, 111
social class, 12
Sofia, 156
Southwark, 27
Sports Council, 66–7
Stanford Heart Project, 111
statistics, 53
Stockholm, 156
Stocking, B., 65–6
strategy, 52
stress, 62, 97–101
stroke, 28–30, 59, 97
suicide, 76, 108

Sustran's, 160
Sweden, 120–1, 125
syringe exchange, 67–8

targets, 23, 24, 70–81, 157–8 and
    Appendix 1
teams, 52
teenage pregnancy, 56–7, 59, 72, 96,
    115–27
Thatchers Britain, 44
therapy, 5, 35, 59
therapeutic era, 18
Thomas, F., 127
tobacco/smoking, 30, 31, 59, 62, 76,
    97–101
Toronto, 69, 131–2, 153, 163
Toronto 2010, 131–2
training, 30
tranquillizers, 104
trends, 1, 42–9, 56–7
true stories, 110, 121–7, 160–1
Turku, 156

underserved groups, 23, 150
unemployment, 10, 67–8, 76, 108
United Kingdom Healthy Cities
    Conference, 165
Urban Adventures, 131
urban regeneration, 160–1
U.S.A., 45–9, 127–32

Vauxhall, 108
vertical programmes, 86–7, 118–20
Vienna, 156
Virchow, R.L.K., 31, 91
VISTA, 130
Voluntary Service Overseas, 129–30
Vuori, H., 58

water, 23, 59, 74, 75, 157
Welsh Heart Project, 111
Wilkinson, Hindle, 107
Womens Movement, 10
work, 30
World Health Organization (WHO), 8,
    21–6, 32, 114, 117, 152–67
world peace, 159

years of life lost, 8
youth, 114–32

Zagreb, 156